HEALTH
INFORMATION
SYSTEMS

HEALTH INFORMATION SYSTEMS

Design Issues and Analytic Applications

—๑

Elizabeth A. McGlynn · Cheryl L. Damberg

Eve A. Kerr · Robert H. Brook

RAND Health

Supported by the John A. Hartford Foundation

The research described in this report was supported by the John A. Hartford Foundation.

Library of Congress Cataloging-in-Publication Data

Health information systems : design issues and analytic applications
    / Elizabeth A. McGlynn . . . [et al.].
        p.   cm.
    "Prepared by RAND Health."
    "MR-967-HF."
    Includes bibliographical references (p. 251).
    ISBN 0-8330-2599-6 (clothbound)
    ISBN 0-8330-2630-5 (paperback)
    1. Health services administration—Data processing.
    2. Information storage and retrieval systems—Medical care.
    I. McGlynn, Elizabeth A.
    RA971.6 .H44   1998
    362.1 ' 068 ' 4—dc21   98-44204
                                                                   CIP

RAND is a nonprofit institution that helps improve policy and decisionmaking through research and analysis. RAND's publications do not necessarily reflect the opinions or policies of its research sponsors.

Published 1998 by RAND
1700 Main Street, P.O. Box 2138, Santa Monica, CA 90407-2138
1333 H St., N.W., Washington, D.C. 20005-4707
RAND URL: http://www.rand.org/
To order RAND documents or to obtain additional information, contact
Distribution Services: Telephone: (310) 451-7002; Fax: (310) 451-6915;
Internet: order@rand.org

ABOUT THE SERIES
DIRECTIONS IN HEALTH SERVICES RESEARCH AND POLICY

This series, focused on the most important analytic and policy issues in health care today, draws on path-breaking research conducted at RAND Health, the nation's largest private health care research organization. Addressing nearly every dimension of the health care system's performance, this work has included innovations in measurement of appropriateness, quality, and health status that have profoundly influenced the field of health sciences research.

Each volume in the series integrates the findings from key studies in the area, then maps the future analytic landscape, highlighting the key questions that both the research and policy communities must address and pointing out the challenges that addressing them will entail.

Series editors are Elizabeth A. McGlynn, Ph.D., Director of the RAND Health Center for Research on Quality in Health Care, and José Escarce, M.D., Ph.D., Co-Director, RAND Health Center on Health Care Organization, Economics, and Finance.

This volume introduces a new series from RAND Health. Focused on the most important analytic and policy issues in health care today, the series draws on the more than three decades of path-breaking research we have conducted on topics touching nearly every aspect of the health care system. By sharing both methodological insights and policy analysis expertise, we further our mission of improving health care systems by advancing understanding of how the organization and financing of care affect costs, quality, and access.

Robert H. Brook, M.D., Sc.D., F.A.C.P.
Vice President and Director of RAND Health

CONTENTS

Part 1
Health Information Systems: An Overview for Policymakers

Part 2
Technical Issues in Designing and Improving
Health Information Systems

FIGURES

TABLES

ACKNOWLEDGMENTS

This book is truly the product of a team effort and the team goes far beyond the editors and individual chapter authors. The John A. Hartford Foundation provided the grant support to develop the material for and write the book. We owe a great deal of thanks to Richard Sharpe who not only had the vision to support the community health data system effort, but gave us the opportunity to participate in providing some of the technical and analytical assistance. We appreciate his perseverance and encouragement throughout the process of writing this book.

We received constructive comments along the way from the various community health data system sites; they continued to encourage us to make the book as concrete and user-friendly as possible.

Eve Schenker was invaluable in tracking down loose ends, reading and commenting on various versions of the chapters, and generally providing excellent research assistance. John Hernandez and Laura Petersen helped develop the Glossary to translate the acronyms, technical terms, and jargon we insisted on including. Mary Vaiana restructured the book to make it suitable for multiple audiences and guided the overall production of the book

An entire team of secretaries was necessary to produce the book: Tamara Majeski was responsible for most of the original typing and coordinating the final product; Patti Sue Titus produced the reviewers' version of the manuscript (including all those last minute changes that each author felt were essential); and Jeri Jackson and Janice Jones were wonderful pinch hitters for bits and pieces of the book. Patricia Bedrosian edited the final volume.

At the beginning of planning this book, we received constructive suggestions and ideas from our colleagues at Value Health Sciences, especially Jackie Kosecoff and Mark Wynn. The book was substantially improved in response to comments from the reviewers, Paula Diehr and Virginia Riehl.

Finally, we have borrowed from a vast literature of textbooks, articles, and some of our own previous work, various ideas, and displays to make the points concrete. We appreciate receiving permission from the authors of these documents to reproduce their work.

AAPCC	Adjusted Average Per Capita Cost
ACG	Ambulatory Cost Group
ACIP	Advisory Committee on Immunization Practices
ACOG	American College of Obstetricians and Gynecologists
AFDC	Aid to Families with Dependent Children
AHA	American Hospital Association
AHCPR	Agency for Health Care Policy and Research
AIDS	Acquired Immunodeficiency Syndrome
AMA	American Medical Association
ANOCOVA	Analysis of covariance
ANOVA	Analysis of variance
ARIMA	Autoregressive integrated moving average
BPH	Benign prostatic hypertrophy
BSA	Blue Shield Association procedure coding system
CABG	Coronary artery bypass graft
CAD	Coronary artery disease
CAPI	Computer-assisted personal interviewing
CAT scan	Computerized axial tomography scan
CATI	Computer-assisted telephone interviewing

CDC	Centers for Disease Control and Prevention
CEO	Chief Executive Officer
C.I.	Confidence interval
COBRA	Consolidated Omnibus Budget Reconciliation Act
COV	Coefficient of variation
CPS	Current Population Survey
CPT-4	Current Procedural Terminology
CRVS (1974)	California Relative Value Scale
CSAQ	Computerized self-administered questionnaires
CSI	Computerized Severity Index
CT	Computerized axial tomography (also CAT scan)
CVA	Cerebrovascular accident
DCG	Diagnostic Cost Group
DHHS	Department of Health and Human Services
DPT	Diphtheria, pertussis, and tetanus
DRG	Diagnosis Related Group
ED	Emergency department
EDC	Estimated date of confinement
EKG	Electrocardiogram (also abbreviated as ECG)
ER	Emergency room
FEHBP	Federal Employees Health Benefits Plan
FFS	Fee-for-service
FIPS	Federal Information Processing Standards
FOBT	Fecal occult blood testing
GDP	Gross domestic product
GHAA	Group Health Association of America

GTE	General Telephone and Electric
HB	Hepatitis B
HCFA	Health Care Financing Administration
HCPCS	HCFA Common Procedural Coding System
HEDIS	Health Plan Employer Data and Information Set
HHANES	Hispanic Health and Nutrition Examination Survey
Hib	*Haemophilus influenzae* type B
HIE	Health Insurance Experiment
HIV	Human Immunodeficiency Virus
HMO	Health Maintenance Organization
HRSA	Health Resources and Services Administration
HS	High school
ICD-9	International Classification of Diseases, Ninth Revision
ICD-9-CM	International Classification of Diseases, Ninth Revision, Clinical Modification
IOM	Institute of Medicine
IPA	Independent practice association
JAMA	Journal of the American Medical Association
KCF	Key Clinical Finding
LMP	Last menstrual period
MAUS	Mammography Attitudes and Usage Study
MEPS	Medical Expenditure Panel Survey
MMR	Measles, mumps, and rubella
MMWR	Morbidity and Mortality Weekly Report
NAMCS	National Ambulatory Medical Care Survey
NBER	National Bureau of Economic Research

NCHS	National Center for Health Statistics
NCI	National Cancer Institute
NCQA	National Committee for Quality Assurance
NHANES	National Health and Nutrition Examination Survey
NHIS	National Health Interview Survey
NHLBI	National Heart, Lung and Blood Institute
NIH	National Institutes of Health
NKAB	National Knowledge, Attitudes and Behavior Study
NMES	National Medical Expenditure Survey
OB-GYN	Obstetrics and gynecology
OME	Otitis media with effusion
OPV	Oral polio virus
PCI	Per capita income
PHS	Public Health Service
PIH	Pregnancy-induced hypertension
PORT	Patient Outcomes Research Team
PPO	Preferred provider organization
PPS	Prospective Payment System
PRUTRAC	Prudential Insurance Company's procedure coding system
PTCA	Percutaneous transluminal coronary angioplasty
PV	Polio virus
QOC	Quality of Care
RBRVS	Resource Based Relative Value Scale
RCT	Randomized Controlled Trial
RUG	Resource Utilization Group

s.e.	Standard error
SES	Socioeconomic status
RAND-36	36-item short form survey developed by RAND to assess an individual's health status
SOII	Severity-of-Illness Index
SSN	Social Security number
Td	Tetanus-diphtheria
TIA	Transient ischemic attack
TURP	Transurethral resection
UB	Uniform Bill
UCSD	University of California, San Diego
US	United States
USC	University of Southern California
USPHS	United States Public Health Service
USPSTF	U.S. Preventive Services Task Force
VLBW	Very low birthweight

This book introduces the basic concepts of health services research—the key policy concerns that shape such research and the specific techniques used to conduct it. The book's central purpose is to provide practical guidance about using different types of data effectively to answer questions posed by a variety of stakeholders in the U.S. health care system.

The book is structured to meet the needs of multiple audiences. For chief executive officers (CEOs) and corporate decisionmakers, it offers a broad overview of the critical issues in using health care data. The book's technical chapters address analytic topics of concern to researchers and analysts who are working in private and public sector groups and are responsible for purchasing, managing, delivering, and regulating health care services.

WHAT DO STAKEHOLDERS WANT TO KNOW?

Stakeholders in the U.S. health care system include private and public purchasers of health plans, physicians, health plans, consumers, and public health programs. Each stakeholder wants access to information for different reasons. For example, private and public purchasers need to decide which health plans to offer their employees and want to ensure that they are getting the best value for their premium dollar. Physicians must keep abreast of advances in medicine so that they can provide full information to patients about treatment alternatives. Health plans need to manage enrollees effectively, monitor contracts with providers and facilities, and make financial decisions. Consumers must select health plans, doctors, and other health professionals that will meet their needs and contribute positively to their health status. Public health programs are responsible for ensuring that the health of the population is maintained and for tracking progress toward established community health goals.

WHAT IS WRONG WITH CURRENT HEALTH SYSTEM INFORMATION?

Many health care decisionmakers share a concern that available health care information is too limited or is of insufficient quality to meet these diverse information needs. The following are among the most important limitations of data from every source:

- Lack of unique identifiers for patients, providers, and facilities, rendering it impossible to track the course of patients' care over time;

- Variation in the quality of data provided, limiting the ability to draw reliable conclusions;

- Lack of uniformity in data elements across data systems, making it difficult to compare patients, providers, and health plans; and

- Lack of important pieces of information required to conduct even the most simple analysis.

The absence of reliable, balanced information about the performance of the health care system has undesirable, and sometimes unintended, consequences. For example:

- **Prices not aligned with costs.** Premiums are based on expectations about the cost of providing services to a population with certain characteristics. If a premium reflects a young, healthy population and policy changes result in large increases in the number of chronically ill enrollees, the premium may not be adequate to provide care.

- **Detrimental effects on health and functioning.** Much of the limited information available about quality of care does not apply to individuals with chronic disease. If health plans that provide good preventive services are less successful in providing care for chronic conditions, and if the available information on quality focuses primarily on preventive health services, individuals with chronic conditions who shift into health plans that provide poor chronic disease care may experience significant and perhaps irreversible declines in their health and functioning.

- **Distorted market for health care plans.** Many purchasers have emphasized cost more heavily than quality in their decisionmaking. But equal attention must be given to developing good clinical indicators of quality. Without such information, excellent health plans that provide care at a somewhat higher cost may be driven out of the market or may choose to compromise the quality of care delivered to meet the cost requirements.

- **Disenfranchised groups with special needs.** Failure to assess what is happening to individuals with rare disorders, those who do not speak English, or those with multiple health problems may result in system changes that leave those individuals without adequate sources of care. Most current monitoring efforts are not appropriately structured to analyze health issues for such groups.

Concerns about poor health care information have stimulated efforts at many levels to build more integrated systems that will provide reliable information to inform decisions. Communities, states, managed care plans, and providers are seeking ways to enhance the quality of information currently being collected, to broaden its range, and to integrate information from a variety of sources to address more complex issues.

Whether such efforts take place in a national health maintenance organization (HMO) or a local hospital, decisionmakers must understand the following core issues:

- What kinds of questions can be answered by a given data source?

- What are the limitations of each source and how they might be overcome?

- Under what circumstances can information from multiple sources be merged, and to what effect?

- What new information would significantly enhance decisionmaking?

Even more basically, those concerned with improving their health care information systems must focus clearly on the kinds of decisions they expect the system to support and the ways the system's results will be used.

In this book, we provide a conceptual framework for addressing both the strategic and the tactical issues involved in integrating and using different types of data to answer a wide range of questions about the performance of the health care system. The framework is applicable to health information systems at any level—individual provider, community, or national entity.

Part 1 presents a policy perspective on health information systems. We profile the data sources, reviewing the kinds of questions each can be used to answer and the limitations and potential enhancements to each source. We provide a high-level view of what a consumer of research needs to know to evaluate and use analyses of health systems data. We conclude by considering evolving national policies regarding performance measurement and the federal government's role in creating a supportive environment for the information systems that will make performance measurement possible.

To maximize the utility of Part 1, we frequently refer the reader to more detailed discussions of key topics appearing elsewhere in the volume.

In Part 2, we examine the analytic enterprise in more detail. We describe the most common sources of data for analysis of health policy issues, with a focus on what improvements are needed to enhance the utility of the data. The chapter on general analytic issues provides a step-by-step approach to analysis and a sampler of some analytic techniques. We review key issues in constructing a clinical data base and provide some concrete illustrations of how to develop such systems. An overview of survey design highlights potential problems and solutions in conducting surveys. We conclude with a review of risk-adjustment issues and techniques.

Part I

HEALTH INFORMATION SYSTEMS

AN OVERVIEW FOR POLICYMAKERS

Chapter One

BUILDING AN INTEGRATED INFORMATION SYSTEM

DATA SOURCES FOR AN INTEGRATED INFORMATION SYSTEM

Integrated information systems, designed to overcome limitations of existing data systems, will draw information from five basic sources:

- **Administrative files:** data generated from an interaction between a patient and provider in the health care delivery system.

- **Enrollment files:** data generated about individuals enrolled in employer-based or government (e.g., Medicare and Medicaid) health insurance plans.

- **Clinical information:** data maintained in medical records, laboratory, or radiology test result systems and from other clinical contacts.

- **Surveys:** data generated from routine or special surveys of individuals about issues such as health status and functioning, health risks and behaviors, and patient satisfaction.

- **Other data:** data collected by various organizations on hospitals, health plans, and other areas of interest (e.g., vital statistics and cancer registries).

A useful way of thinking about potential uses of integrated data networks is captured in the matrix below (Table 1.1), which illustrates how data from these sources intersect with the generally accepted dimensions by which health care system performance is measured: *access*, the freedom and equality of opportunity to obtain adequate and effective health services (Aday et al., 1993); *cost*, the combination of health goods and services that produces the maximum benefit for society within a set budget (Aday et al., 1993); and *quality*, the degree to which health services for individuals and populations increase the likelihood of desired health outcomes and are consistent with current professional knowledge (Lohr, 1990).

Table 1.1

A Data Matrix

Sources of Data	Dimensions of Performance		
	Access (Equity)	Cost (Efficiency)	Quality (Effectiveness)
Administrative			
Enrollment			
Clinical			
Survey			
Other			

For example, reading across a row in the matrix, administrative data can be applied to answer questions about access to health care services, cost of health care, and quality. Additional data make it possible to answer increasingly sophisticated and complex questions.

Table 1.2 illustrates the increasing complexity of questions that can be answered with the addition of different data sources. Administrative data alone allow one to construct fairly crude measures of access—the number of procedures paid for. The addition of enrollment data, such as age and gender, allows one to construct access rates for the entire population and facilitates making adjustments to a standard population so that rates can be compared. The addition of clinical data, such as the extent and location of blockage in the coronary arteries and prior treatment history, allows one to assess whether the

Table 1.2

Integrated Information Systems Facilitate Answering More Complex Questions

Data Source	Research Question	Purpose
Administrative	How many coronary artery bypass graft (CABG) surgeries were paid for last year?	Access
Administrative + enrollment	What was the age-adjusted rate of CABG surgery among men and women?	Access
Administrative + enrollment + clinical	What proportion of CABG surgeries were done for clinically appropriate reasons?	Quality
Administrative + enrollment + clinical	What is the risk-adjusted mortality rate following CABG in different hospitals?	Quality
Administrative + enrollment + clinical	What is the risk-adjusted price of CABG in different hospitals?	Efficiency
Administrative + enrollment + clinical + survey	Do patients return to normal functioning at different rates depending on the hospital that did the surgery?	Efficiency

procedures were clinically justifiable. These data also allow one to risk-adjust outcomes such as mortality so that different entities can be compared fairly. These risk adjusters also help in the evaluation of efficiency. Adding patient survey data can allow one to understand efficiency from a broader perspective, such as return to functioning.

Table 1.2 also illustrates that the area in which the question is being asked may dictate the type of data needed. For example, most administrative data do not include clinical detail adequate to answer questions about the technical quality of care delivered. Similarly, answers to questions about patient functional status will require a survey in which individuals are asked directly for their assessments.

WHAT KIND OF DATA SHOULD AN INTEGRATED INFORMATION SYSTEM INCLUDE?

Among the first decisions confronting those planning integrated information systems are the kinds of data to include in the system and the priorities for building its various components. In both cases, the decision depends on the expectations one has for the system, the type of information most needed by key decisionmakers, and the ways in which the results will be used. The following questions provide a general framework for thinking about these issues:

- What questions do stakeholders want answered?

- When do those stakeholders need answers?

- What are the consequences of acting on inaccurate information?

What Questions Do Stakeholders Want Answered?

One can gather useful information about the questions stakeholders want answered by asking representatives of stakeholder groups to generate a set of questions for which they feel they need answers to accomplish their role effectively. At a minimum, these groups should include consumers, health care providers, health plans/payors, policymakers, employers, and researchers.

An effective way to elicit this information is to convene focus groups—a small number of individuals from a stakeholder community brought together under the leadership of a facilitator to collectively develop a list of key questions. The interactive nature of focus groups often produces a richer set of questions than might be generated if individuals were queried separately. Convening groups with similar backgrounds may provide a freer exchange of ideas.

Gathering information from stakeholder groups is more than just a consensus-building process. Various groups may share an interest in a general topic but want to ask very different questions about the topic. The ways in which those questions vary will have important implications for the data required. To illustrate this point, consider the example of childhood immunizations (Table 1.3).

In this example, the substantive area of concern is the quality of preventive services, specifically, the provision of age-appropriate immunizations. The shared subgroup is children under age two, which suggests that one needs information on the birthdate of children to identify the right group for analysis. More specific data elements can be identified by examining the questions posed by each group:

- Consumers have framed the question in terms of health plans in their community, which implies the ability to produce plan-specific rates of immunization (i.e., link children to health plan).

- Providers are interested in how they might increase rates of immunization, so they need a link between rates of immunization and different methods for ensuring that children receive this service (e.g., reminder systems).

- Health plans are interested in whether they are missing opportunities to immunize children; this requires being able to produce utilization profiles for children in this age group and to explore whether children who are not receiving immunizations are getting other services, during which time they could also have been given an immunization.

- Policymakers are interested in knowing immunization rates at the community level, which requires linking children to geographic areas (e.g., by zip code).

Table 1.3

Illustrative Set of Questions Posed by Different Stakeholders

Stakeholder	Question
Consumer	Last year, which health plan in my area had the highest rate of up-to-date immunizations for children under age two?
Provider	What strategies have worked well for other providers to increase the rate of childhood immunizations?
Health plan	Are we missing opportunities to immunize children who present for other types of health care?
Policymaker	Did providing free immunizations at the local health clinic in Anytown last year improve the rate of immunizations in that community compared to the prior year?
Employer	Last year, which health plan provided our employees with the highest rate of up-to-date immunizations for children under age two?

- Employers are interested in how well services are being delivered to their employees, which requires identifying children within health plans linked to a specific employer. Although many employers may accept information about overall health plan performance, some may want to know if their employees are receiving services at the same rate as others in the health plan.

For most of the questions posed by stakeholders, the time frame is at a single point in time (e.g., the most recent year for which data are available). However, the policymakers' question requires two points in time—before and after implementation of a public health program. The providers' question implies a comparison between using and not using a mechanism for increasing immunization rates (e.g., reminder cards for parents).

Asking stakeholders what they are interested in knowing about the health care system can help shape the strategy for developing an effective integrated information system—one that serves the needs of the widest group of potential users. The example above illustrates the slightly different data needs of groups asking questions about the same general area of concern. If only one of these groups had been queried, the data base might be missing a key variable required to answer questions posed by another group.

When Do Stakeholders Need Answers?

One motivating force behind developing integrated information systems has been the difficulty of producing information for decisionmakers in "real time," that is, within the time frame required by the decisionmaking process. Both new data collection and analysis of existing data require a considerable investment of time and expertise. As a consequence, by the time an answer is developed, the decision may already have been made or the information may be out of date. For example, if a patient is facing heart surgery, three-year-old hospital mortality data may not be indicative of the quality of care the patient is likely to experience today.

Consider what timeliness might mean in the context of the three major functions of integrated information systems.

Data Repository. In its role as a data repository, the integrated information system serves the widest potential set of users and purposes; each of these users and purposes will imply different time requirements for the data.

- Consumers who want information to make health plan choices will need information that is current and available during their open enrollment period (e.g., on an annual basis).

- Primary care providers who are making referrals to specialists will need information that is current and available on-line. Presumably they would prefer to be able to query the system to individualize the referral (e.g., by geographic location, expertise in a particular disease or procedure, gender, or race) to meet the needs of the patient.

- Health plans may be interested in comparing their performance to that of other health plans and will need information for designated time periods.

- Policymakers may need information to make quick responses to legislative proposals or during budget deliberations. This will require the ability to quickly produce customized analyses in response to specific questions.

The availability of data through integrated information systems will almost surely increase the demand for such information and raise expectations about the currency of the information and the ease with which data can be accessed. Therefore, those responsible for maintaining these improved health care data systems should consider setting standards about the timeliness with which data are made available to different user groups. These standards can be reviewed over time to evaluate whether they are adequate and meet the evolving needs of the system's users.

Information Sharing Network. Sharing information requires rapid availability of data—for example, transmitting laboratory results directly from the laboratory to the physician. For many tests, rapid communication of laboratory results would be extremely valuable and would reduce the delay in treatment for patients who have serious diseases (e.g., cancer).

Transaction Processing. The expectation for any integrated data network is that transaction times will not increase from current levels and should be as rapid as possible. The technology is available to ensure that the eligibility of an individual to have a claim paid can be checked as the claim is submitted; at the same time, the completeness of the claim form can be evaluated and claims with incomplete information can be rejected.

What Are the Consequences of Acting on Inaccurate Information?

A critical concern in planning, building, and maintaining an integrated information system is whether the information it contains will be accurate enough to be used in a decisionmaking process. Examples of the kind of information that can be misleading highlight the importance of this concern:

- The first time the Health Care Financing Administration publicly released information on mortality rates by hospital, it did not take into account the relative levels of illness among patients at admission. Thus, some of the hospitals that had the "worst" rankings were those primarily serving a terminally ill population. Subsequent releases controlled for severity of illness profiles of patients. Similar severity-adjustment strategies will be necessary to compare a variety of performance measures.

• When the Pennsylvania Health Care Cost Containment Council releases information on the mortality rates from coronary artery bypass graft surgery by individual physician, it does not provide data on physicians who performed fewer than 30 procedures annually, because the numbers for those doctors would not be statistically meaningful. Taking into account whether differences are statistically significant is important, because it indicates when the differences could not have occurred simply by chance.

• Many surveys have low response rates—in some cases only 20 percent of people who are sent questionnaires return them. It is frequently the case that those who return questionnaires are different in important ways from those who do not return questionnaires. Drawing conclusions on the basis of only those who returned questionnaires could lead to erroneous decisions. For example, if individuals who are satisfied with their health plan are less likely to return questionnaires, an employer could conclude that a health plan was doing poorly with company enrollees and might decide not to offer that plan a contract next year.

WHEN IS EXPERT HELP REQUIRED?

For any step in the development and use of integrated information systems, the individuals and groups responsible for directing the effort may require expert consultation. Examples of the types of experts who might be consulted are shown in Table 1.4.

Table 1.4

Illustrative List of Areas of Consultation and Experts

Potential Consultation Area	Type of Expert
Defining stakeholder questions	Focus group facilitator
Deciding on data elements for issues related to	
Costs of health care	Economist
Access to health care	Health services researcher
Quality of care	Physician
Organization of services	Organizational behaviorist
Patient satisfaction	Psychometrician
Insurance coverage	Economist
Developing clinical data bases	Physician
	Biostatistician
	Health services researcher
	Medical records technician
	Nurse
Conducting surveys	
Survey design	Survey research specialist
	Psychometrician
Sampling	Statistician
Fielding surveys	Survey research specialist
Analysis	Health services researcher
	Statistician
	Economist
	Clinician
	Computer programmer

Chapter Two

DATA SOURCES FOR AN INTEGRATED INFORMATION SYSTEM

In the previous chapter, we identified five basic sources from which integrated information systems could draw and considered how data from each source can be used to answer different kinds of questions about the health care system. In this chapter, we consider these data sources in more detail, with special emphasis on identifying their current limitations and suggesting improvements.

Many of the data sources discussed in this chapter are public use files, available on-line. In Chapter Five, where more technical aspects of the data sources are presented, we provide the relevant Web addresses.

ENROLLMENT DATA

Enrollment data are generated by employers and individuals. The primary purpose of these data is to identify those eligible for coverage under a particular insurance plan, private or public.

Uses of Enrollment Data

Payors (health plans and the government) use enrollment data to determine whether they are authorized to pay a claim.

Analysts use enrollment data to ask a wide range of questions about the performance of the health care system. For example, at what rate do either certain conditions or specific treatments occur in the population of enrolled persons? Comparison of such rates provides a way to gauge differences in health plan performance. However, so that plans or hospitals are rated fairly, these measures must be adjusted for differences in the characteristics of the groups of enrollees. As a consequence, it is essential that enrollment data capture information such as age and gender, which can be used for risk adjustment (discussed in Chapter Nine).

Enrollment data are also extremely useful for addressing questions such as which groups have unmet health care needs, how treatment outcomes differ across population subgroups, and which geographic areas merit more resources. Morbidity, mortality, access to care, utilization of services, and health behavior all vary by age, race, gender, and socioeconomic status (i.e., income and education). Enrollment data are a good source of this kind of information, which is typically missing from administrative or clinical data records.

Problems with Existing Enrollment Data

Existing enrollment data typically have important limitations. Understanding these limitations and possible improvements increases the utility of these data sets for analysis.

Not all files are routinely updated. Each insurer or health plan determines how frequently its eligibility files will be updated, and the frequency varies considerably. Some insurers, such as managed care plans, require that employers provide information every month about which employees are covered under the health plan. In fact, the plans are frequently paid an amount for each member for each month enrolled (called, "per member per month"). In contrast, some indemnity plans collect eligibility information at the time of initial enrollment but update this only annually or when an employer submits a change of status form for the worker (e.g., when employment is terminated). The net result is that enrollment data vary widely in currency and, therefore, in the extent to which they accurately reflect the true population enrolled in or covered by a health plan.

At a minimum, users of enrollment data should inquire about the frequency with which files are updated so that they understand the data's potential limitations in accurately defining the population eligible to receive health services. In addition, users may not be able to compare data from sources with different rules for updating. These concerns are especially germane to the Medicaid population, whose eligibility for enrollment in the insurance plan varies from month to month.

Important information may be missing. Enrollment files may be lacking important information, such as the total number of subscribers on a policy, their ages, and their relationship to the insured. This information is necessary for many analytic purposes, including sampling (e.g., identifying all insured individuals with certain cost-sharing requirements); calculating rates of certain procedures, such as immunization; and adjusting utilization rates for age.

In addition, because enrollment files are based on insurance status, anyone who resides in the community and who is uninsured or not covered by a government program is not included in these files. Analysts must use different strategies—for example, surveys—if they wish to describe population-based rates of service, such as influenza immunization.

Enrollment files lack sufficient detail and uniformity. The contents of enrollment files reflect that their function is to determine eligibility for coverage. As a consequence, the data may lack details such as the enrollee's health status—a piece of information analysts need to assess adverse selection among health plans or for risk-adjusting other performance measures. Such gaps are exacerbated by the fact that each insurer requests different pieces of information on enrollees, with a consequent lack of uniformity across different enrollment files.

Changes that would make enrollment data more useful for evaluation and quality-monitoring purposes include the following:

- Requiring insurers to update files regularly;

- Developing greater uniformity in the information collected; and

- Expanding the set of variables to capture more information germane to health care utilization, costs, and outcomes.

ADMINISTRATIVE DATA

Administrative data are generated as a result of a patient's encounter with a health care provider—physician, hospital, pharmacy, laboratory, and radiology facility.

Uses of Administrative Data

Insurance companies and other payors generally use administrative data to pay bills and manage operations. These data are typically computerized, making it easy to collect and use large quantities of information.

Policymakers, employers, and health plans have used administrative data for a variety of purposes, including to monitor changes in the health care system. For example, administrative data have been used to examine geographic variation in utilization of surgical and medical procedures, monitor the use of health services, assess the effects of a policy change on health expenditures, compare how different cost-sharing arrangements affect use of medical care, and evaluate the relationship between hospital death rates and hospital characteristics.

Problems with Existing Administrative Data

Administrative data have certain limitations that make them less useful for secondary applications.

Use of diagnosis and procedure codes varies. Often, different diagnosis (International Classification of Diseases, ICD-9-CM) and procedure (Current Procedure Terminology, CPT-4) codes can be used to describe the same event. Thus an analyst trying to compare costs, treatment processes, or outcomes for a disease across different doctors, hospitals, or health plans may find that different types of patients are included in these comparisons.

Diagnosis codes tend to encompass broad ranges of disease severity and, therefore, may mask important clinical subgroups that differ in their expected response to treatment. In addition, diagnosis codes do not allow analysts to determine an individual patient's severity of illness, often a necessary step in interpreting analytic results. Instead, this information must be obtained from the patient's medical record, usually by manually abstracting the information—a costly and time-consuming procedure.

Accuracy and completeness of coding are not consistent. The accuracy of diagnostic coding can vary substantially across hospitals and physicians. Although some of the observed differences may be due to human error, others may reflect responses to financial incentives.

For example, the financial incentives provided by Medicare's Prospective Payment System (PPS) improved the completeness and accuracy of coding because reimbursement is contingent upon complete coding. But PPS also provided hospitals with a financial incentive to code conditions to maximize reimbursement (referred to as "upcoding"). As a result, the primary diagnosis coded may be the one that ensures the highest payment and not the condition that is the most clinically salient or the primary condition for which the patient sought treatment.

Timing of diagnoses is uncertain. The diagnostic information that appears on claims forms makes it impossible to distinguish between a condition that arises during the course of treatment (a complication) and a condition that was present at the time the patient was admitted to the hospital (a comorbidity). Being able to make this distinction is essential for judging the quality of care that the patient received. Without knowing the timing, one might inappropriately classify a condition that existed before admission as a complication of care received while in the hospital or incorrectly conclude that the hospital performed poorly because of the "complication" when, in fact, the patient had the condition when admitted.

The presence of other medical problems and the sequences of clinically important developments are generally more accurate when obtained from clinical data. If clinical data were routinely available, the combination of clinical and administrative data would significantly expand the potential analytic uses of both these files.

Key information on test results is lacking. Test results provide critical information about the diagnosis and treatment of medical conditions—information that is essential for evaluating quality of care. But test results are not generally available in administrative files because they do not affect the reimbursement rate, the establishment of which is the primary function of the administrative data system.

In the current environment, the analyst must obtain test results from the patient's medical record or perhaps from an automated laboratory test system that includes results. Medical record abstraction is relatively expensive and few automated test result systems exist that are linked to other data systems.

No information exists on those who have not used the health care system. Only individuals who have contact with the health system produce an administrative record; healthy individuals, or those who are ill but do not seek treatment, are not included. Similarly, in health systems where a claim must be filed for an individual to be reimbursed, the administrative files will not contain information about services for which a claim was not submitted—for example, if the amount of the service is small or less than an individual's deductible. As a consequence, relying on administrative data alone could result in undercounting the actual number of individuals with illnesses and, in the case of healthy persons, overestimating rates of use of preventive services.

Ways to improve administrative data include

- Developing a common set of operational definitions for diagnostic and procedure codes;

- Showing payors and providers how to improve coding practices;

- Requiring coding of diagnoses that captures information on all existing conditions;

- Conducting periodic coding audits to improve quality;

- Incorporating core clinical data elements that facilitate severity adjustment; and

- Establishing unique identifiers for patients, hospitals, and physicians so that information from separate sources can be linked.

CLINICAL DATA

The medical records maintained by hospitals and physicians are the most common source of clinical data. These records contain information on a patient's medical history, primary complaints, presenting symptoms, physical examinations, clinical assessments and diagnoses, diagnostic test results, procedures performed, medications, response to treatment, the clinical course of the patient, discharge plans, and demographic factors such as age, gender, and race. The medical record describes what occurred from the clinician's perspective. All of this information is confidential, and special permission is required to gain access to it.

Uses of Clinical Data

Because clinical data contain the actual diagnostic information, they can be used to study the extent to which medical and surgical procedures are appropriate, the quality of care performed by providers and health plans, the clinical outcomes for particular procedures or treatments, and the access of certain groups to specific types of care.

For example, a purchaser could use clinical data to compare two health plans on a selected set of performance measures, such as adequacy of blood pressure control or appropriateness of coronary artery bypass graft surgery. Because clinical data contain risk factors—for example, the patient's principal diagnosis and the presence of comorbid conditions—the analyst can adjust for severity of illness, thus "correcting" for differences in patient characteristics or health risks that may influence the outcome of care, independent from medical treatment.

Problems with Existing Clinical Data

Like other data sources, clinical data have their limitations and problems.

Patients may have multiple records. In some systems, each patient may have multiple medical records because a new medical record is established each time the patient seeks care from a different doctor or hospital. Thus, to get a complete picture of the care a patient received for a medical condition, an analyst would need to obtain the patient's medical records from several sources.

Patients lack unique identifiers. Like administrative and enrollment data, clinical data do not contain a unique individual identifier for each patient that is common across all health care facilities or delivery systems. This lack makes it difficult to link clinical data to other data sources for more comprehensive analyses.

Records lack standard format. Medical records have no standard format or procedures for recording information and often vary considerably in how information is recorded. For example, some clinicians may note the presence or absence of symptoms or medical history elements whereas others may make a notation only when symptoms or history items are present.

Because there is no uniformity in what clinicians are required to document in a patient's medical record, information may be missing or may vary in how it is presented, rendering uniform comparisons difficult. For example, the information in the medical record might not be complete enough to explain why two patients with similar medical conditions received different treatment.

Data are difficult to obtain and assess. Medical records are not generally maintained in a form suitable for analytic purposes. Currently, when detailed clinical information about a set of patients is required for a study, the data have to be manually abstracted from the records after care has been delivered. (From the information on the abstraction forms, researchers construct data elements or variables.) Most medical records exist only in paper (hard copy) format, and most entries are hand written. As a consequence, abstracting information from these records is costly and time-consuming. In addition, the information in the records is highly variable and requires interpretation (e.g., whether the absence of a note on smoking means that the patient does not currently smoke or that the physician did not ask whether the patient smokes).

Data have subjective elements. Medical record information reflects both the subjective evaluation of the provider and objective results from clinical tests. Clinicians may differ among themselves on the diagnosis, severity, and recommended course of treatment for the same patient, or they may forget to record information in the clinical record. As a result, analysts must consider all the possible reasons why information needed for analysis may not have been included in the clinical record and what these gaps may imply for drawing conclusions from the data.

Many health care providers are moving toward entering clinical data at the time of service into an automated system. This prospective, computerized data collection would

- Make clinical data available more quickly;

- Provide opportunities to prompt clinicians for more data on certain types of conditions or patient factors that may relate to treatment outcomes; and

- Promote greater uniformity in the information available to evaluate clinical performance.

Chapter Seven provides a detailed discussion of enhancing the collection of clinical data and improving its accessibility and utility.

SURVEY DATA

Survey data are most often used to study special issues or populations not captured in the routine data collection systems described above.

Uses of Survey Data

Surveys of health plan enrollees or patients can generate person-level information on issues such as patient satisfaction with care, functional and health status, quality of life, health habits, and usual source of care.

Surveys of providers can enhance understanding of the type of services provided, the type of patients seen, knowledge of clinical practice guidelines, and providers' satisfaction with their current practice.

Surveys are conducted by a variety of groups, including health plans, business coalitions, employers, provider associations, consumer advocacy groups, and local, state, and federal governments. Surveys can be annual, ongoing, periodic, or one-time only. Users of survey data should obtain the survey's documentation, which describes the sampling method used, a copy of the survey as fielded, and names and definitions of data elements.

Problems with Survey Data

Surveys are expensive. Surveys can be expensive (especially when conducted correctly) and are generally done only when an important question arises that cannot be answered from other data sources. Patient satisfaction surveys are an example.

The survey's "time perspective" drives results. The majority of surveys are designed as cross-sectional studies (i.e., the survey is conducted one time only). As a result, they allow evaluation only of what is occurring at a given point in time. Cross-sectional data can produce results that vary significantly from longitudinal data (i.e., surveys that capture information on the same people over a longer period of time). For example, the estimate of the number of Americans uninsured at a given point in time differs from the estimate of how many were uninsured at any time during the year.

Survey results are hard to interpret correctly. The results derived from a survey may be difficult to interpret correctly for various reasons; for example, the sample drawn from the population may not be representative, or there may be low response rates or poor recall on the part of respondents. If those who respond to the survey differ in important ways from those who did not respond, the survey results will not provide accurate answers to the questions being asked.

Survey data usually lack unique identifiers. As a general rule, surveys do not contain linking variables designed to facilitate merging survey data with other information on the respondent. Indeed, to protect the confidentiality of respondents, unique identifiers such as social security number or medical record number—as well as other identifiers that could be used for linking purposes, such as name, address, zip code, or state—are usually removed from the file before the data are made publicly available. Exceptions are surveys conducted by health plans that want to link survey data to clinical data maintained on persons enrolled in the health plan (e.g., to assess functional status after treatment for a hip fracture). Such exceptions require informing respondents that such linkages and uses of data are planned.

Information produced by surveys may not be timely. Survey data may take a long time to collect and analyze. As a consequence, the information surveys produce may not be very timely. A number of technical issues also affect the quality of all surveys. These include ensuring a sufficiently large number of responses, appropriately matching the persons to whom the survey is given with the group of interest, and knowing how to handle missing data. These and other technical issues involving surveys are discussed in Chapter Eight.

OTHER DATA SOURCES

Many other data sources are available from state and federal governments as well as from private groups. Several of the more important include

- Birth certificates;

- Death certificates;

- Birth defects registries;

- Disease registries (e.g., cancer and end stage renal disease);

- Provider characteristics; and

- Facility characteristics.

These data files are very useful for studying the health care system—for example, tracking health outcomes or monitoring changes in the incidence and severity of diseases over time.

As with every type of data that we have considered, the most critical issue related to using these other sources is the ability to link records at the level of the patient or provider. In their current incarnation, these data sources do not contain unique patient or provider identifiers that are commonly applied across data systems. Many may require special permission for use in analyses other than those for which the data were originally obtained. For example, some states require that the mother's permission be obtained to use data from birth certificates.

STRATEGIES FOR IMPROVING THE UTILITY OF INTEGRATED INFORMATION SYSTEMS

The limitations of the data sources described above hamper analysts' ability to gain maximum value from the health information currently available. Moving toward maximally useful information systems will require addressing the four overarching issues shown in Table 2.1. The table also suggests measures that data system managers could take to begin addressing these issues.

FOR MORE DETAIL

In Chapter Five, we describe these data sources in more detail and, when possible, give the Web addresses for public use files. Chapter Six touches on issues that arise in using these data for analysis. Chapter Seven describes enhancements to a clinical information system. In Chapter Eight, we consider various aspects of surveys, including design options, sampling methodology, the characteristics of cross-sectional and longitudinal designs, and the details of implementing a survey.

Table 2.1

Improving the Utility of Integrated Information Systems

Problem	Recommended Actions
Lack of unique identifiers for linking purposes	Establish unique identifiers for each patient, health care provider, and health plan/payor to be used in all data bases Evaluate opportunities to make the identifier consistent with federal coding schemes, such as the Medicare facility ID, to achieve broader linking ability To ensure adequate protection of privacy, establish procedures for who will have access to identifying information and under what conditions Design a system to issue and monitor the use of unique identifiers
Uneven data quality	Establish operational definitions for assigning diagnosis and procedure codes and disseminate the definitions to providers and payors Require full (five-digit) coding of diagnosis codes to distinguish differences in severity of illness/condition Conduct periodic audits to assess accuracy of coding in encounter data; compare against clinical data Provide financial incentives to encourage complete and accurate coding Set priorities and a timetable for automating clinical data
Lack of uniformity of data elements across different data systems	Identify those data elements for which standardization across all payors and providers of care is critical Establish common definitions and coding conventions for these data elements Develop interface systems to facilitate comparability Provide financial incentives to ensure the use of uniform coding on standardized data elements
Missing data elements	Review existing data forms to determine what is collected and what important elements may be missing Build consensus among policymakers, payors, providers, and consumers about the data elements that should be added Revise forms/collection instruments to include those items

Chapter Three

WHAT CONSUMERS OF RESEARCH NEED TO KNOW ABOUT ANALYSIS

What does a consumer of research need to know when requesting analyses of data or examining the analytic results of others? In this chapter, we address this question by reviewing some of the basic steps in any analysis. We will use childhood immunizations as an extended example because it illustrates a broad range of issues that might be analyzed using the information contained in health system data bases.

FORMULATING THE QUESTION

Analysis begins with formulating a question to be answered. The more specific the question, the easier it will be to develop an answer. For example, the very broad question, "What proportion of people in the state received needed preventive services?" lacks, among other things, a definition of needed services, a target population (the population to whom the answer applies), a time frame, and any indication of how often services should have been rendered.

We can make this question easier to answer by providing a time frame, specifying a target population, giving an explicit indicator on which performance will be measured, and identifying a single type of preventive service. For example:

> During calendar year 1998, what proportion of children under age two were up-to-date on their immunizations?

We could refine the question further by limiting the evaluation to a geographic area or to selected subgroups (e.g., by race/ethnicity, low-income households, type of vaccine, or type of health insurance).

Here are some issues to consider when defining the research question.

Who is the primary audience for the answer? For example, an employer interested in knowing how well the health plans with which it contracts are doing in immunizing children might wish to compare immunization rates experienced by its employees' children with those of other children enrolled in the health plan. In contrast, if a state health department is asking the question, the population to whom the answer applies—uninsured and insured children—might be quite different.

Why is the question important?   We expect analytic questions to generate information that leads to action. For example, questions that probe whether certain groups have problems obtaining certain health services might lead to programs that improve access to needed services.

How will the answer be used?   The answer to a question must generate enough information to support a decision. For example, if a state discovers that a portion of its children are not being immunized, it needs to know if those children are evenly distributed across the state's population or concentrated in certain subgroups.

DESIGNING THE STUDY

Conducting analyses based on existing (secondary) data poses certain challenges. Because the analyst cannot alter the design of the original study, he or she must understand how the design will affect the kinds of analysis the data will support and the kinds of conclusions that can be drawn from the analysis. Sometimes, the analyst can choose between different data sets, produced by different study designs, each with its own advantages and limitations.

Figure 3.1 gives a simple illustration of the choices made in study designs and the resulting study classification.

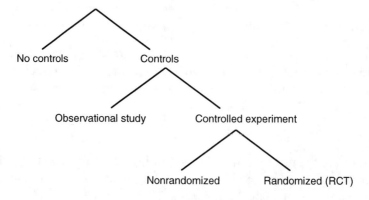

SOURCE: Adapted from Freedman et al. (1978).

Figure 3.1— General Classification Scheme for Study Designs

Often, the effectiveness of an intervention or treatment is tested by comparing a patient who received it (a member of the "treatment" group) to one who did not (a member of the "control" group). Studies that do not have control groups do not provide much useful information. Because there is no basis for comparison, there is no basis for concluding that a given outcome is the result of the treatment.

Individuals can be assigned to the treatment or control group in a variety of ways. The basic question is, Does the investigator decide who is assigned to the control group? If the answer is yes, then the study is a "controlled experiment." If it is no, then the study is an "observational study."

Bias is an inherent problem in observational studies because participants may choose which group to participate in. For example, people who already have healthy life styles may be more likely to participate in a study testing the effect of vigorous daily exercise. However, in some cases, ethical or practical concerns make an observational study the only option. For example, we cannot randomly assign people to "smoker" and "nonsmoker" groups to study the effects of smoking on health. Some of the biases associated with observational data can be removed in analysis.

If the study is a controlled experiment, the basic question is, Are individuals randomly assigned to the control and treatment groups? If the answer is yes, then the study is a randomized controlled trial, often abbreviated as RCT. Because such studies guard against bias by leaving group membership to chance, they are regarded as the gold standard in empirical research.

Random assignment can happen in several ways. For example, in a double-blind placebo RCT, neither the investigator nor the patient knows which group any of the participants have been assigned to. Or randomization may be stratified—that is, certain groups (e.g., all female or all children under age 12) may be randomized separately.

The pool of participants available for random selection may also be formed in various ways. The pool might be formed over a particular time period—for example, all patients who receive treatment in a particular hospital in a given month. Or a control group could be chosen historically—for example, patients who visited a particular hospital in the year before a certain treatment was in use. Other ways of forming control groups are used when the outcome of interest is rare and finding cases is difficult.

When a control group cannot be formed, an individual may function as his or her own control. In this "pre-post" design, measurements are taken before and after an intervention and compared. Pre-post designs are limited in terms of the inferences that they will support because of the number of changes that can occur outside of the study that influence its results.

The time at which the comparison groups are constructed is also important. In prospective studies, the comparison groups are defined, then followed forward in time. In retrospective studies, the groups are defined, then measurements are constructed by looking back at historical data. In general, prospective studies are less subject to bias.

Studies can be cross-sectional or longitudinal. In the former, whether the individual received the intervention and its outcomes are both measured at a point in time. In a longitudinal study, whether the individual received the intervention is usually measured before measuring the outcomes, and several outcome measurements may be taken over time. Longitudinal studies provide a stronger basis for drawing conclusions.

The advantages and limitations of various study designs are discussed in more detail in Chapter Six.

IDENTIFYING THE DATA SOURCE

Chapter Two described a variety of data sources available in the health system. Deciding which of these sources to use requires determining which data are likely to produce the most accurate answer or contain the most complete information, then weighing that determination against the relative cost of obtaining data from each source. A common aid for matching questions with appropriate data sources is a *data dictionary*—a catalogue of what information is available from different data sources.

We illustrate the use and combination of various types of data by considering the data necessary to answer the above question about childhood immunizations.

The population who should be immunized can be identified through *enrollment data.* Information about those in this group who actually received immunizations can be obtained from *administrative*, *clinical*, or *survey data*— either singly or in combination. The performance indicator (whether immunizations are up-to-date) can be determined by referring to existing standards of care as recommended either by the U.S. Public Health Service (PHS) or from an appropriate specialty society (e.g., the American Academy of Pediatrics).

To answer the question, information must be linked at the level of the individual across multiple sources. Linking raises a number of issues. For example, the children identified as being in the correct age range using the enrollment data must be identical to those for whom immunization rates are examined, using administrative, clinical, or survey data.

In this example, three possible data types—administrative, clinical, or survey—could be used to provide information about which children have received immunizations. What is the best source to use?

There may not be one "correct" answer. For example, survey data are more likely to capture the child's immunization experience across different service providers (e.g., health plan, county health department, or school clinic) but are affected by whether the parent remembers accurately which immunizations were given and on what date.

In selecting data sources, one must always trade off ease of use, accuracy, content, and purpose of analysis. Each choice requires different techniques to optimize the data's utility in answering the study question. Knowing the data's limitations allows the analyst to make the most of the information available. The strengths and weaknesses of key health system data sources, as well as suggestions for improving them, are discussed in detail in Chapter Five.

CONSTRUCTING THE ANALYSIS FILE

Having identified the sources of data to answer the question, the next step is to construct the analysis file—that is, assemble in one file all the data elements or observations needed for the analysis. Doing this requires making a series of decisions discussed briefly below. In our discussion, we focus on data that already exist (often called secondary data because they were originally collected for a purpose other than the current one).

Restricting the File to a Subset of Individuals

For many analyses, the starting point will be to identify characteristics of individuals on whom the analysis will be conducted (e.g., the target population). These characteristics might include age, geographic location, insurance status, time frame, a specific disease, and so on.

It may be desirable to further limit the number of persons in the analysis file by selecting a sample of eligible individuals. Simple random sampling (i.e., all eligible individuals have an equal probability of being sampled), which is easily accomplished by a computer, is the preferred technique for selecting a sample. Any deviation from it should be adequately justified by a statistician.

Statistical techniques called precision and power calculations help determine how large the sample should be to obtain useful estimates and to compare subgroups in a meaningful way. (These techniques are discussed in more detail in Chapter Six.) These calculations might include relatively more of certain subgroups in the analysis file (called oversampling).

Selecting Variables

The analysis file should contain only the variables required for the study. Variables can be either

- **Dependent variables:** the outcome of interest or event that you want to understand (e.g., whether a child is immunized); or

- **Independent variables:** factors that influence or are related to the dependent variable (e.g., the child's ethnicity, whether the child lives in a rural or urban area, and the child's health insurance status).

For example, to answer the childhood immunization question, three types of variables could be constructed from the various data sources:

1. **Individual characteristics,** such as date of birth, gender, race/ethnicity, and geographic location, can serve as independent variables for the analysis. This information can be obtained primarily from enrollment data, supplemented by and linked in some cases to administrative and clinical data. Including information about individual characteristics allows the analyst to examine whether differences in the rates at which children are immunized are related to sociodemographic characteristics.

2. **Characteristics of the health system** are also independent variables. This information, obtained from surveys, helps the analyst understand whether aspects of service delivery either promote or inhibit timely immunization. This information might also be found in data bases that maintain information at the facility level.

3. **Immunization indicators** serve as dependent variables. Information about the provision and timing of each type of immunization allows the analyst to construct the pattern of service for each child. Immunization indicators might be obtained from administrative, clinical, or survey data.

Catalogues of variables (data dictionaries) for each potential data set make it much easier to construct an analysis file. In particular, if the variable the analyst wants to use is not in the data base, he or she may need to create a new variable from existing ones or substitute another variable. The catalogue will greatly simplify this process.

Merging Data from Different Sources

Because analyzing immunization rates requires information from more than one source of data, the data sources will have to be merged to create a single record for each individual. How to merge the data depends on the focus of the analysis. For example, a focus on individuals suggests choosing a unique individual identifier as a merging variable. As noted above, such identifiers are not widely used today because of privacy concerns. If the analysis focuses on information about institutions, then the identifier for the hospital, health insurance plan, or other institution may be the most appropriate merging variable.

When unique identifiers are not available, merging data sources becomes substantially more difficult. The analyst must turn to other identifiers that are not unique but provide for relatively high rates of matching (e.g., name, date of service, and date of birth).

Without a unique identifier, linking data sources to explore common questions about the delivery and cost of health care can be time-consuming and expensive. (Chapter Six provides an example.) In addition, linking files without benefit of a unique identifier requires special care to prevent biases of unknown magnitude or direction from being introduced.

Initial Data Quality Checks

Once the analytic data set is assembled, the analyst will assess the quality of the data to identify problems that might affect the results of the analysis. Typical steps in a data quality check include the following:

1. **Checking for common data problems:** This step includes, for example, looking for entries that are out of the possible range or entries that are not internally consistent. The analyst will have to develop decision rules about how to deal with inconsistent data.

2. **Addressing problems of missing data:** The analyst must determine, for example, why data are missing, whether the missing data can be ignored (and with what consequences for the results), or if statistical techniques should be used to fill the gaps.

3. **Identifying errors in measurement, both random and systematic, and selecting an approach to deal with bias in the sample on which the analysis will be based:** Random errors are less problematic because they tend to offset each other when measurements are averaged. Systematic errors must be adjusted for because they can introduce bias into the data and thus result in inappropriate conclusions being drawn from the analysis. Adjusting for bias

usually requires consultation with a statistician. Various approaches to dealing with bias are described in Chapter Six.

SELECTING AN APPROPRIATE ANALYTIC TECHNIQUE

Selecting an analytic technique depends on the study design, the questions to be answered, and the type of data available. Generally speaking, analysis falls into three major categories:

- **Descriptive:** This category involves examining data in tabular, graphical, or numerical form to identify important patterns in the data. Descriptive analysis is the first step in any analysis and provides a context within which other information can be considered.

- **Inferential:** This involves drawing conclusions about a population beyond the one that was included in an analysis.

- **Predictive:** This technique involves using information to estimate future results.

The results of both inferential and predictive analyses contain some level of uncertainty because our conclusions are based on information drawn from a sample rather than from the entire population. However, the degree of uncertainty in an inferential or predictive analysis can be measured and stated quantitatively.

Chapter Six discusses the major analytic techniques in detail, gives examples of their application, and discusses appropriate ways to use inference and prediction. Chapter Six also provides a list of suggested references (see Table 6.22)

INTERPRETING THE RESULTS

The final stage of an analysis is considering its implications and deciding what actions should be recommended. In general, this involves answering the following kinds of questions:

1. **Do the results make sense?** This question must be answered in the context of what people have found in prior studies and what appears to happen in the real world. It is vital to check all possible reasons why the results of this analysis should differ from previous studies or are counterintuitive. There may be good explanations, but they must be found and carefully considered.

2. **Is the result statistically significant or meaningful?** This involves computing a test to assess whether the result is due to a real effect or to chance.

3. **Is the result important?** What difference would it make if someone acted on the study results? Answering this question requires looking at the size of the effect. There is no absolute rule for making this determination: It depends on the specific problem. A small change may be very important if it affects a large number of people—for example, even a slight change in the use of services by the Medicare population could have enormous cost implications. In contrast, a large change that affects only a small group may have a limited effect—for example, a large change affecting only those with a very rare illness will have a small overall effect.

4. **What should be done next?** For example, a decisionmaker might decide to further analyze the data, to examine a new question identified in the analysis, to implement a policy change and monitor its effect, or to reevaluate the same question in the future.

FOR MORE DETAIL

The use of unique identifiers to link files is described in Chapter Five. Analytic techniques and ways to identify and deal with bias are discussed in Chapter Six. Issues associated with surveys are addressed in Chapters Five and Eight.

Chapter Four

THINKING STRATEGICALLY ABOUT INFORMATION SYSTEMS

In the last five years, the debate about the performance of the nation's health care system, once almost exclusively focused on costs and utilization, has broadened to include concern for increasing the value (quality) for health care dollars spent. Information systems are at the heart of monitoring the quality of care. Financial and organizational strategies can be blunt and clinically insensitive in their applications, and both needed and unneeded care can be eliminated as cost controls are introduced. In the absence of quality monitoring, we cannot determine whether cost-control efforts are compromising quality. Thus, quality monitoring is an important tool for making optimal resource allocation decisions.

The National Committee for Quality Assurance (NCQA) (1997b) issued a clarion call for the development of information systems that will provide data making it possible for purchasers and health plans to make choices based on value, not just cost. Describing the measurement of the quality of health care as "one of the most critical challenges of coming years" but "primitive" compared to the assessment of the quality of other goods and services, the report provides a road map to communicate "directly to the managed care industry what upgrades in information systems will be necessary" to increase their ability to measure performance, thus creating an environment in which "advanced performance measures can be implemented at a reasonable cost" (p. 6). The report includes both immediate and longer-term initiatives.

The NCQA urges health plans to improve the use of currently available data over the next two to three years, by improving its quality; create an environment that rewards automating clinical information; position themselves to implement new standards; improve their current data-management practices; establish policies for protecting confidentiality; and begin to plan for the cost of expanding, updating, and replacing their current software, hardware, and communications technology to meet new information requirements.

In three to five years, the NCQA suggests, a number of likely developments will make it possible for health plans to implement new information systems that meet the full demands of performance measurement. These changes include federal standards for structure, contents, definition, and coding of the elements of a medical record; federal legislation to protect privacy; vendor software that automates patient records in compliance with standards; and communication technology that makes sharing of clinical data possible.

Bringing about these changes requires support from other organizations, in particular the federal government. If these developments do not take place, health plans will have to continue their own efforts to improve their information capacity.

While acknowledging that the challenges of implementing new information systems are formidable, the NCQA is developing performance measures that assume "the implementation of its road map recommendations in the timeframe specified."

The centrality of enhanced information systems in the nation's future health care system as well as the federal role in creating a supportive environment for them are highlighted in the report of the President's Advisory Commission on Consumer Protection and Quality in the Health Care Industry.

> Health care information systems of the 21st century must be able to guide internal quality improvement efforts; generate data on the individual and comparative performance of plans, facilities, and practitioners; help improve the coordination of care; advance evidence-based health care; and support continued research and innovation (p. 213).

Noting that existing information systems are not adequate for these purposes, the commission recommended a number of actions intended both to spur and to coordinate efforts to address these inadequacies. The recommendations include

- Encouraging investment in information systems by having purchasers of health care services insist that providers and plans be able to produce quantitative evidence of quality;

- Incorporating health care information systems, including automation of clinical information, improvement of data quality, and participation in regional or national health information networks, among the standards used by quality oversight organizations;

- Establishing national standards for structure, content, definition, and coding of health information;

- Implementing security programs to protect confidentiality;

- Making use of information technology in clinical settings a part of training health care professionals; and

- Supporting demonstration projects designed to illustrate and test improvements in information systems.

Both the federal government, through the Quality Interagency Coordinating Committee, and the private sector, through the Forum for Health Care Quality Measurement and Reporting, are working to implement the recommendations of the Advisory Commission. With respect to information systems, a key concern is that addressing the potential problems associated with computer handling of dates in the next century (known as the Y2K problem) is absorbing all resources that might otherwise be used to improve health information systems.

There may be consensus about what we want and need health information systems to do in the 21st century, but as the NCQA report notes, many issues remain unresolved. The federal government, health care organizations, and foundations must collaborate to explore issues such as the effect of automation on the quality of patient care, the costs and benefits of computerized patient records, the effects of automation on provider work flow and productivity, the development of data input methods and technology that are adapted to the patient care process, and the requirements for structured medical language that is compatible with both the delivery of care and the discipline of information systems.

Part 2

TECHNICAL ISSUES
IN DESIGNING
AND IMPROVING
HEALTH INFORMATION
SYSTEMS

Chapter Five

DESCRIPTION OF DATA SOURCES AND RELATED ISSUES

by Cheryl Damberg, Eve A. Kerr, and Elizabeth A. McGlynn

INTRODUCTION

A variety of data sources might be used to address questions of interest to consumers, purchasers, regulators, physicians, and health system managers. A few examples demonstrate how integrated health data systems could potentially be used:

- To help consumers select health plans and providers of care in their geographic area based on cost and quality performance;

- To enable doctors and hospitals to improve the quality of the care they provide to patients;

- To facilitate the establishment of high-quality, cost-effective provider networks by insurers and employers; and

- To permit state and federal health agencies to track, over time, the effect of policy changes on the public's health.

Although individual data sources can be used for a range of analyses, mechanisms for combining and integrating data across various sources create opportunities for more powerful and meaningful analyses. Such integration of sources has been proposed at the community or state level and some integration has occurred with individual delivery systems. Each source of data has limitations that also should be addressed to improve the quality of the information that can be derived from it. This chapter has three major purposes. First, it provides a brief introduction to each data source. Second, it highlights some of the current limitations of each source. Third, it identifies issues that must be addressed to enhance data source integration efforts. Wherever possible, we have provided sources and Web addresses for publicly available data.

DATA SOURCES: EXISTING SYSTEMS

Data currently collected and used by decisionmakers to examine the functioning of the health care system can be broadly classified as coming from five sources: (1) administrative files, (2) enrollment files, (3) medical records, (4) surveys, and (5) other data files.

In broad terms, each of the five data sources currently serves a specific function, such as reimbursement for services rendered or eligibility determination for insurance coverage. Consequently, the data elements contained in each serve to support the underlying function of that data base. However, the sources also contain information that can be used to evaluate a variety of issues related to the performance of the health system. Table 5.1 illustrates how several of the data sources can be useful for different types of studies.

The following subsections describe the five core data sources, including potential uses, function and design, data elements, characteristics of ideal data bases of each type, problems with current data sources, and ways to evaluate the quality of a data set.

Administrative Data

Definition. Administrative data are generated as a result of a patient encounter with a health care provider, including ambulatory (outpatient) care, hospital services, and pharmaceuticals. Data are generated by both health professionals and facilities. Sometimes these data are referred to as "claims" or "encounter" data; claims data are usually generated to pay claims, whereas encounter data are generated to track the number and content of visits in capitated systems. Insurance companies and other payors, such as the government, collect and maintain this information for reimbursement and other administrative purposes. Administrative data are typically computerized, which facilitates their use in analysis because large quantities of data are available. As a result, policymakers, employers, and health plans have used administrative data for a variety of purposes, including to monitor changes in the health care system.

Potential Uses. Table 5.2 illustrates various ways in which administrative data could be used to answer certain types of questions about health care utilization, costs, and the outcomes of treatment. The footnotes give examples of studies that have been conducted using these data. However, as is discussed below, administrative data have a number of limitations that can hinder their utility for these purposes.

Function and Design. The primary function of administrative data is to support reimbursement activities in noncapitated or indemnity health plans (e.g.,

Table 5.1

Characteristics of Data Sources for Different Types of Information

Issue/Study Area	Clinical Data	Patient Report (Survey)	Administrative Data
Access to care	May be able to assess access to necessary care	Provides both subjective and objective assessments	Data on frequency of visits only
Use of services	Data may need to be obtained from several records	Dates and content of care subject to recall problems	Best source for covered services; unreimbursed care not represented
Symptoms	Recording will reflect doctor's assessment of importance	Most inclusive source	No information on symptoms
Interpersonal aspects of care	Rarely recorded	Best source for patient perspective	No information
Technical aspects of care	Data available on most important processes	Patients may be good reporters, but recall of content of past visits varies	Adequate if eligible population can be identified and criteria reflect a billable service provided
Diagnostic tests	Good source, particularly for test results	Patients recall testing in general terms, but may not know specific results or types of tests	Good source of data for whether tests are done, although test results not generally available
Medications	Good source for prescription drugs; over-the-counter drugs may not be recorded	Fair source of information on current medications	Good source for prescription medications filled by participating pharmacy or claim filed
Patient education	Detail often lacking	Patients can report on what they understood	Only available if reimbursable and coded separately
Outcomes of care	Useful for biological outcomes, but data on other outcomes, such as functional status, are often missing	Richest source of data on patient functional status	Useful for assessing mortality and other selected outcomes likely to be recorded on claims
Expenditures	Useful for identifying individuals with specific conditions to evaluate costs of treatment	Data likely to be affected by recall	Primary source of cost data

SOURCE: Adapted from Siu et al. (1991).

Table 5.2

Illustrative Uses of Encounter Data

Utilization studies
  Monitor the use of health services over time
  Study geographic variation in the utilization of surgical and medical procedures[a]
  Identify providers with unusual practice patterns[b]
  Track referrals to specialists
  Compare the use of surgical procedures by age, race, or gender for a specific health condition[c]

Cost studies
  Evaluate the effect of utilization review and utilization management programs on costs[d]
  Assess the effect of a policy change on annual health expenditures (e.g., addition of a new health benefit or expanded provision of services)
  Measure differences in the cost of services among types of health plans[e]
  Compare the effect of different cost-sharing arrangements on the use of medical care[f,g]

Outcomes evaluation
  Assess the effect of a policy change on health outcomes[h,i]
  Evaluate differences in hospital death rates as a function of differences in the quality of care[j]
  Examine readmissions to hospitals within a specified period after surgery[k,l]

SOURCES: [a]Wennberg (undated); [b]Welch et al. (1994); [c]Ayanian and Epstein (1991); [d]Wickizer (1990); [e]Newhouse et al. (1985); [f]Anderson et al. (1991); [g]Newhouse and the Insurance Experiment Group (1993); [h]Haas et al. (1993); [i]Piper et al. (1990); [j]Park et al. (1990); [k]Roos et al.(1987); [l]Wennberg (1987).

fee for service (FFS) or Independent Practice Association (IPA)). In contrast, capitated managed care plans do not routinely generate administrative data because reimbursement is on a per-member rather than a per-service basis. As a consequence of its reimbursement function, existing administrative data often do not contain the specific variables, the level of detail, or the quality control that are required to evaluate clinical issues or policy changes. For example, demographic and health status information on enrollees in a health plan typically is not captured in administrative data because this information is not required by the insurer to pay the bill. Today, if you wanted to examine the relationship between health status and resource use (e.g., medical expenditures), you would need to obtain data on health status from another source (e.g., a survey). However, administrative data do not use a consistent set of identifiers (i.e., social security number or subscriber number) so linking administrative data to other data sources with different identifiers is more difficult. Integrated health data systems could solve this problem by providing either a uniform identifier or the necessary linkages to enable users to extract information from a variety of data sources and to assemble the different pieces of information for each patient in one analysis file. Integrated health data systems could also enhance existing enrollment data collection efforts to capture health status information on individuals. Taking this step will allow studies to be done that today are either not possible or very difficult to accomplish.

Administrative data are currently collected and maintained by Blue Cross and Blue Shield health plans, some managed care plans, commercial insurers, and the Medicare and Medicaid programs. Each health plan and commercial insurer uses a different data collection form to capture payment information related to hospital care and outpatient care. In addition, each insurer typically has its own unique form to capture information on the clinical encounter, which is then used to process medical claims for health plan enrollees. Because each insurer maintains a different system for processing medical claims, these data are currently difficult to combine to evaluate what is occurring at the community or state level regarding access to care, utilization of services, and costs of treatment.

To illustrate this point, if you wanted to compare the inpatient cost and utilization experience of patients enrolled in different health plans, you would need to combine the administrative files from different insurers (see Box 5.1).

BOX 5.1

ILLUSTRATIVE PROBLEM WITH INCONSISTENT ADMINISTRATIVE DATA

Problem: Large employers in the United States typically contract with multiple health plans to provide coverage for their employees. In response to large cost increases in the 1980s, employers wanted to monitor the cost and utilization experience of their entire workforce to see what was driving costs and whether opportunities existed to control costs. However, employers lacked the ability to evaluate the medical cost and utilization patterns across their entire employee population because each carrier maintained a separate administrative data base that could not be combined with the files of other insurers.

Solution: In response to the growing demand by employers to understand the cause of rising costs, several private companies developed products/systems that would integrate the administrative files from different insurers. Similarly, integrated data systems could facilitate the merger of administrative and other types of data files.

Combining data from different sources is extremely difficult to accomplish in the current environment where each insurer collects a slightly different set of variables, may use different definitions for variables, and may have different ways of coding variables. Specifically, not all insurers use the same diagnosis coding scheme.[1] Prudential uses "PRUTRAC" diagnosis codes that do not map

---

[1] Examples of the various diagnosis and procedure coding schemes used by different insurance companies include International Classification of Diseases, Ninth Revision, Clinical Modification

to the ICD-9-CM codes used by many other insurers. Other carriers have their own unique diagnosis coding schemes that do not match either ICD-9 or PRU-TRAC codes. Because you may want to study the cost or use of care by classes of diagnoses, it is important that diagnoses be coded in an identical manner by all carriers. An additional problem with diagnosis codes in administrative data is that they may be used by physicians to mean either a confirmed or suspected diagnosis, particularly for visits related to evaluating new symptoms. In the administrative data set, one generally cannot distinguish these "rule out" diagnoses from final diagnoses, which can create considerable inaccuracy in data analysis.

Other data elements that tend not to be uniform across all insurers are procedure codes, the type of service units (i.e., days, visits, or procedures), discharge status, outpatient service type, discount reason, provider discount amount, and coverage type (e.g., Preferred Provider Organization (PPO) or HMO). Charge and payment information also varies from insurer to insurer, making it difficult to determine which insurers have negotiated discounts. Insurers often maintain their own set of identifiers for patients and providers that may prevent linking files from various insurers to assess how the delivery of care for a single provider (e.g., a hospital) may vary as a function of the type of payor (e.g., Medicaid or private insurance). Integrated health data systems, on the other hand, must address the issues of data linking and standardization. At the conclusion of this chapter, we summarize a set of actions that would improve uniformity of these data sources and linking across sources generated by different entities.

Data Elements. One of the most widely used forms for submitting hospital claims for payment is the Uniform Bill or the UB-92. The federal government uses the UB-92 to process all claims for Medicare beneficiaries. The UB-92 contains patient and provider identifiers (which are specific to each medical facility); patient name, address, birth date, gender, marital status, admission date and status, and insurance coverage; charge and billing data; diagnosis and procedure codes; admission and discharge date; payor; insurance group number; physician identifiers; and employer name. Other hospital claims forms that private insurers use parallel the UB-92 in terms of general content. Table 5.3 lists data elements that are common to most hospital claims forms.

The federal government uses a standard form, the HCFA 1500, to capture billing information for all outpatient (ambulatory) care visits. The data elements captured by the HCFA 1500 include payor identifier; patient name, address, date of

---

(ICD-9-CM), CPT-4, HCFA Common Procedural Coding System (HCPCS,) 1974 California Relative Value Scale (CRVS), Prudential Insurance Company's procedure code system (PRUTRAC), and 1981 Blue Shield Association procedure coding system (BSA).

birth, gender, and telephone number; insurance coverage with policy number; date of encounter; illness; date and place of service; procedure code; description of services and supplies; charges; amount paid; physician Social Security or tax identifier number; and the dates of service. Table 5.4 lists data elements

Table 5.3

List of Standard Data Elements: Hospital Claims Forms

Patient characteristics
    Patient identifier (unique to each hospital or care facility)
    Name (last, first, middle initial)
    Address (street, city, state, zip code)
    Date of birth
    Gender
    Marital status

Provider characteristics
    Hospital/facility identifier (unique)
    Physician identifier (unique only for Medicare claims)
    Diagnostic and treatment information
    Admission date
    Admission status
    Admitting diagnosis code
    Condition code
    Diagnosis code
    Description of service
    Service date
    Service units
    Principal and other diagnoses (up to 6)
    Principal and other procedures (up to 5)
    Date of procedure
    Emergency code

Insurance/payment information
    Insurance group number (differs for each health plan)
    Group name
    Insured's name
    Relationship to insured
    Employer name
    Employer location
    Covered period
    Treatment authorization codes
    Payor
    Total charges
    Noncovered charges
    Prior payments
    Amount due from patient
    Revenue codes
    HCPCS/rates

SOURCE: HCFA, UB-92 inpatient encounter form
(www.hcfa.gov/medicare/edi/edi5.htm).

captured on the HCFA 1500, many of which are similar to data elements on outpatient claims forms used by private insurers for their own enrolled populations.

Table 5.4

List of Standard Data Elements: Outpatient Claims Forms

Patient characteristics
  Patient identifier—Social Security number or other identifier
  Name (last, first, middle initial)
  Address (street, city, state, zip code)
  Date of birth
  Gender
  Marital status
  Telephone number
  Other health insurance coverage

Provider characteristics
  Physician identifier—tax identifier or other plan-specific identifier
  Physician's employer identification number

Diagnostic and treatment information
  Date of encounter
  Illness
  Emergency
  Admission and discharge dates
  Diagnosis or nature of illness
  Diagnosis code
  Place of service
  Date of service
  Procedure code
  Description of services and supplies
  Date patient able to return to work
  Date of disability

Insurance/payment information
  Payor identifier (e.g., Medicare or Medicaid)
  Group name
  Insured's name
  Insured's identification number
  Insured's group number
  Address and telephone number of insured
  Relationship to insured
  Employer name
  Employer location
  Covered period
  Treatment authorization codes
  Accept assignment
  Total charges
  Amount paid
  Prior payments
  Balance due

SOURCE: HCFA 1500 outpatient encounter form (www.hcfa. gov/medicare/edi/edi5.htm).

Because the principal use of administrative forms is reimbursement on a per-service basis, certain types of managed care plans (e.g., staff model HMOs) do not use such forms. Enrollees pay a set amount (capitation) each month that covers all services used. Many of these organizations claim that their ability to offer comparable services at a lower price than traditional systems is due to the savings in administrative costs from not having to process claims forms for each service or procedure. For a variety of reasons, there has been increasing pressure to have capitated plans incorporate encounter forms (sometimes called "dummy claims") in routine practice as a means to capture greater detail on utilization patterns within the health plan.

In the current claims-processing environment, each private insurer maintains its own unique outpatient claims form. Although these forms are generally similar in content to the HCFA 1500, they can differ in important ways. Some variables appear similar, but coding practices vary widely across insurers. The problem with having multiple, nonstandard claims forms is that the data elements contained in one carrier's claims form are identical neither to those contained in the HCFA 1500 nor to those contained in the claims files of other private insurers. Because of the lack of standardization across health insurance plans of specific data elements, how they are defined, and how they are coded, the process of constructing a unified file from multiple sources is difficult, time-consuming, and expensive. Building a single analysis file is necessary if you want to examine expenditure data from all private health insurers in a state to see whether the expenditures on services varied and if the variation was related to the type of health plan. In making a transition to integrated health data systems, efforts need to focus on ensuring uniformity of a core set of data elements across the administrative data files maintained by different payors. Achieving this goal will facilitate analyses of cost and utilization across health plans, providers, and patients.

BOX 5.2

DEFINITION OF RELIABILITY AND VALIDITY

Reliability: This requires consistency in the results of a measure, a tendency to produce the same results multiple times, and reproducibility of the measure under varying conditions of survey administration. Example (of inter-observer reliability): Would different physicians examining the same patient for a condition assign the same diagnosis code to that patient's condition?

Validity: This requires accuracy of the measure and its ability to reflect the concept. Example: Does a procedure code measure only preventive care (e.g., mammography screen) or does it also include diagnostic services?

Characteristics of an Ideal Administrative Data Base. Administrative data have the advantage of capturing information on a large number of individuals, systemwide; however, these data currently have certain limitations that must be addressed to develop a high-quality, integrated data system. Table 5.5 lists a set of characteristics that define an ideal administrative data base. As the following discussion reveals, existing data do not meet these standards.

Table 5.5

Characteristics of an Ideal Administrative Data Base

Ability to link administrative information to other data files (enrollment and clinical data) on patients, providers, and health plans

Accurate and complete diagnosis and procedure data

Periodic audits to verify accuracy of diagnosis and procedure coding

Data elements that permit a distinction between comorbid conditions and complications associated with treatment

Standard coding of core data elements by all providers and payors

Problems with Existing Administrative Data. Because problems with existing administrative data sources affect the kinds of questions that can be asked and the validity of conclusions that can be drawn, these problems are worth solving. We provide a brief description of some of the most important problems that arise when using administrative data.

Varying reliability and validity of diagnoses and procedure codes. For many procedures and diagnoses, different diagnosis (ICD-9-CM) and procedure (CPT-4) codes can be used to describe the same event. The lack of operational definitions for ICD-9-CM diagnostic codes tends to result in highly variable assignment of codes to health conditions. From a data user's perspective, this makes it difficult to extract all relevant cases within a particular diagnosis code category to examine questions about the costs or patterns of care for a particular condition. For example, bronchitis and upper respiratory illnesses may be coded using different ICD-9-CM codes but may refer to the same condition.

Coding of procedures may also be less precise than is required to answer clinical questions. For example, the coded procedure may not contain a coding extension (a fourth- and fifth-digit modifier) to distinguish whether the procedure was a repeat procedure and, if repeated, whether it was performed by the same or another physician.

Diagnosis codes tend to encompass broad ranges of disease severity and therefore may mask important clinical subgroups that differ in their expected response to treatment. Also, diagnosis codes do not allow direct determination of the patient's severity of illness. A measure of severity is important to control for differences that may affect the observed outcome. For example, hospitals that treat sicker patients would be expected to have higher mortality rates. If the severity of patient illness is controlled for, a high-quality hospital with a large number of very sick patients may have mortality rates similar to those in a lower-quality hospital with less sick patients. Today, to assess severity of illness often requires obtaining data from the patient's medical record. This is difficult to do, since it involves manually abstracting information from the medical record. An integrated clinical data base that captures detailed administrative, financial, and health information on each patient overcomes this problem.

Reporting and coding errors. The accuracy of diagnostic coding can vary substantially across hospitals and physicians. For example, some providers may code a condition or procedure that would not otherwise be reimbursed (e.g., a mental health problem or substance abuse) as a condition or procedure that is covered under the health plan. Because reimbursement amounts for hospital stays are tied to the patient's diagnosis, the accuracy of these codes may be somewhat better than is the case for outpatient encounters where reimbursement is not tied to diagnosis codes. The financial incentives provided by PPS reimbursement have improved the completeness and accuracy of coding, since reimbursement is contingent on complete coding. Although this was a favorable outcome, hospitals also were provided a financial incentive to code conditions in ways that would maximize reimbursement (referred to as "upcoding"). In some cases, the primary diagnosis may be the diagnosis that ensures the highest payment and not the condition that is the most important clinically or the primary condition for which the patient sought treatment. The financial incentives for physician payment under the Resource Based Relative Value Scale (RBRVS) also provide physicians with financial incentives to upcode or to select a medical service or procedure code (e.g., CPT-4) that reflects a higher level of service than was actually performed.

Inability to determine the timing of diagnoses. Since diagnostic information appears on administrative forms, it is impossible to distinguish complications that arise during the course of treatment from comorbid conditions that are present at the time the patient is admitted to the hospital. For example, a patient might develop pneumonia while in the hospital. The record of the hospital stay will indicate the presence of pneumonia, but you will be unable to determine whether the patient was admitted with that condition or whether the condition developed during the hospital stay. Knowing when certain conditions occur during the hospital stay is important for making judgments about the quality of care received by the patient. Without knowing the timing, you might inappropriately classify a comorbid condition that existed before admission as a complication of care that was received while in the hospital.

Timing is also important for adjusting for differences in patient risk that may influence health outcomes, independent of the treatment provided. In the example, you might incorrectly conclude that the hospital performed poorly because of the "complication" if the patient had the condition before being admitted to the hospital. This example underscores the importance of being able to link administrative data to clinical data that document the existence and duration of comorbid conditions.

Lack of information on test results. Although administrative data may account for the fact that a certain event occurred (laboratory test or x-ray), the results of these tests are not generally available in the claims file. This is because the test results do not affect the reimbursement rate, which is the primary function of the administrative data system. Test results are generally found in the medical record although automated laboratory test results systems are becoming more common. These latter systems, however, may be maintained separately by laboratory vendors and may not be routinely linked to other health system data. Such linking is a time-consuming and costly task to perform in the current, nonintegrated data environment. Test results provide critical information on the diagnosis and treatment of medical conditions, which is essential for evaluating the quality of care provided.

Lack of information on nonusers of the system. Administrative records exist only on individuals who have contact with the health system. Relying solely on administrative data to estimate the number of individuals with specific illnesses may result in erroneous conclusions about access to care for persons with certain conditions. Because administrative data do not capture information on healthy individuals—those who never use the system—evaluating the use of preventive services such as screening mammography, childhood immunizations, and Pap smears using this data source alone may overestimate rates of provision of preventive services (i.e., if nonusers are not included in the denominator). If you wanted to compare the characteristics of "nonusers" to "users" you would need to link administrative data to enrollment data that contain all potential users.

Evaluating the Quality of Data. Because the problems just described can affect the quality of an analysis and the accuracy of conclusions, before proceeding with any analysis you should evaluate the quality of the administrative data you intend to use. The following check list (Table 5.6) identifies a series of questions that you should ask before proceeding with an analysis of an existing data source. Chapter Six provides more detail on the methods you can use to test the quality of your data. Table 5.7 offers some suggestions for improvements for those who are responsible for creating and maintaining administrative data files.

Table 5.6

Checklist for Evaluating the Quality of Administrative Data

Do unique identifiers exist to permit you to link administrative data to other data files, by patient, provider, or payor? If not, what variables can be used to link data files (e.g., name or address)?

What proportion of the diagnosis and procedure codes have missing or incomplete data?[a] What analytic strategies should be used to address these missing data problems?

What proportion of the coded diagnoses and procedures are valid? Has this been evaluated in the data base you are using or in similar data bases? What biases will likely occur if data validity is a problem?

Are any of the services to be evaluated typically billed as a single global or flat fee (e.g., maternity care)? How will this affect analysis of utilization patterns?

Do different payors/health plans have different data collection forms and do they differ with respect to which data elements they collect? If so, how can these be reconciled?

Are data elements commonly defined and coded by all insurers and providers who produce administrative data? If not, how will data files be constructed?

---

[a] If more than 5 to 10 percent of all medical claims are missing codes or have incomplete codes, you should be concerned about bias in your results if you analyze these data. (See Chapter Six for more information on bias.) At a minimum, you should seek to identify differences between complete and incomplete records to determine if those cases with missing data occur randomly (e.g., some from each provider) or in a systematic way (e.g., all from one health plan or hospital).

Administrative data are a valuable resource for evaluating the performance of the health system. To improve the utility of these data sets for analyses, entities that currently maintain these systems should consider how best to incorporate the recommendations in Table 5.7 into their existing systems. Collaboration among entities at the national level to institute these recommendations consistently and comprehensively would maximize the value of these data sets for a variety of analyses.

Table 5.7

Steps for Improving the Quality of Administrative Data

Develop a common set of operational definitions for diagnostic and procedure codes.

Educate payors and providers on how to improve coding practices.

Require full five-digit coding of diagnoses (ICD-9-CM) to capture information on comorbid conditions.

Conduct periodic audits to compare diagnosis and procedure codes to information contained in the medical record and provide feedback to health plans and providers for quality improvement.

Begin to identify the core data elements that should be included in a clinical data system.

Establish unique identifiers for patients, hospitals, and physicians to enable the linking of files.

Enrollment Data

Definition and Function. Enrollment (or eligibility) data are generated by employers and individuals for use by health plans and the government (the payors). The primary function of enrollment data is to identify the group of persons who are eligible for coverage under a particular insurance plan, be it private or public. Payors use these files to determine whether they are authorized to pay a claim.

Uses of Enrollment Data. Enrollment data are critical for answering even the most basic questions about the health system, since they define the population of individuals who are eligible to receive care by a health plan. The primary function of enrollment files from an analytic perspective is to identify the population about whom questions will be asked. For example, enrollment files can be used to construct age-adjusted rates of procedure use, to construct samples for surveys, and to identify cases for medical record review.

By knowing the total number of individuals eligible to receive care and the number of people who actually received care (from administrative or clinical data sources), you can compute and compare the rates at which diseases or treatments occur in the population of enrolled persons—such as the cesarean section rate, the rate of coronary artery bypass graft surgery, the complication rate associated with receiving a surgical procedure, or the mortality rate. These measures provide one way to gauge differences in health plan performance. To allow a fair comparison between health plans, these measures would need to be adjusted for differences in the health risks of the groups of enrollees. Therefore, it is also very important that enrollment data capture information that can be used for risk adjustment, such as age and gender. (See Chapter Nine for a detailed discussion on severity and risk adjustment.)

Enrollment data can also serve as an important source of demographic, employment, and health plan information that is not generally captured in administrative or clinical data records. Because morbidity, mortality, access to care, utilization of services, and health behavior vary by age, race, gender, and socioeconomic status (i.e., income and education), this type of information is extremely useful for understanding where unmet health needs exist, how treatment outcomes differ across population subgroups, and where to target resources. Thus, enhancing the type of data captured in enrollment files offers an important opportunity for improving data systems.

Data Elements. The basic data elements contained in an enrollment file include the name and address of the policyholder, the coverage type (family or single policy), an employee identifier (unique to the worker's own firm),[2] the employer's name and address, a group insurance policy number, the effective date of coverage, the policyholder's date of birth, and in some cases the policyholder's Social Security number. Often, separate identifiers are not used for the employee and her or his dependents. Enrollment files also rarely contain information on whether the enrollee has dual coverage (e.g., from a working spouse). Enrollment files vary in the data elements contained in the files (see Table 5.8). For example, some insurers require information on only broad coverage classifications (single, two-person, or family), which means that they do not capture actual counts of the number of eligible beneficiaries or person-level data about those who are covered.[3] Other insurers require the names and relationships to the policyholder of each person covered under the plan, as Table 5.8 illustrates. With this level of detail about enrollees, you could determine the actual number of people covered under the plan, which is extremely important for calculating rates of service provision (e.g., immunization rates and hospital admission rate). If you do not know the number of people in the health plan, you cannot accurately determine what proportion of the enrolled population is using services.

Table 5.9 lists data elements typically found in an enrollment file. It should be noted that the specific data elements vary by employer and health plan. Requiring a uniform set of data elements for each health plan would enhance the utility of these data sets for a variety of analytic purposes.

Table 5.8

Example of Enrollment File for Company A

Policyholder	Type of Coverage	Others Covered	Relationship to Policyholder
Jane Doe	Family	John Doe	Husband
		Beth Doe	Child
Ted Smith	Family	Sally Smith	Wife
		Tina Smith	Child
		Jeb Smith	Child
		Jack Smith	Child
		Katie Smith	Child
Susan Jones	Single	—	—
Jack Kane	Two-person	Dana Kane	Wife

---

[2]An individual who holds more than one job and is covered under two employers' health plans would have two employee identification numbers in the enrollment files.

[3]In this case, only information contained in the second column of Table 5.8 would appear in the enrollment file. Note that family sizes can vary.

Table 5.9

Data Elements Common Among Enrollment Files

Employee information
  Name of policyholder (first, last, middle initial)
  Address (street, city, state, zip code)
  Coverage type (single, two-person, family)
  Individual policy number (unique for each carrier)
  Social Security number
  Date of birth

Employer information
  Employee identifier (unique for each business)
  Employer name
  Employer address
  Group insurance number (unique to the insurer)
  Effective date of coverage for policyholder
  Coverage dates for all other covered persons
  Consolidated Omnibus Budget Reconciliation Act (COBRA)
    coverage (yes or no)

Limitations in Using Enrollment Data. There are limitations associated with using enrollment data that analysts need to take into account. First, enrollment files vary in how often they are updated, with the frequency of update determined by each insurer or health plan. Some insurers, such as fee-for-service plans, require monthly updates from employers on who is covered under the health plan. Mid- and large-size employers provide the insurer with monthly eligibility tapes that are generated from payroll information. In contrast, some health plans collect eligibility information at the initial time of enrollment and the data are updated only when an employer submits a change of status form for the worker (e.g., some HMOs). This issue is especially germane to the Medicaid population, whose enrollment in the insurance plan varies from month to month. Medicare beneficiaries can also change health plans once a month. Most persons covered under employer-sponsored insurance plans are restricted to making changes once a year. If infrequently updated, enrollment data may be unreliable for determining the true population of insured persons who are eligible for coverage. Also, because frequency of updates varies by employer, combining several enrollment files for an analysis may result in a noncomparable data set.

Second, important information may not be included in the file, such as the total number of dependents on the policy, their ages, and their relationship to the insured. Not having separate records for each eligible person makes it difficult to determine the total number of covered persons. For example, it is very common for insurers to estimate an average number of dependents per policy depending on whether the policyholder selects single or family coverage. This estimate is used to calculate the number of covered lives in a health plan so that insurers can set premiums, and for this purpose, averages work sufficiently well. However, this approach does not provide an accurate count of the number of individuals who are insured, which is necessary for other analytic uses. Similarly, the lack of demographic information on additional covered persons (i.e., gender and age) limits the use of enrollment data for sampling and other analytic activities (e.g., calculating rates of immunization among children under age two or calculating mammography rates among women over age 50).

Third, because enrollment files are designed to define who is eligible for coverage under a given insurance plan for reimbursement purposes, the data do not always provide the level of detail required for many of the most basic health care analyses, such as the enrollee's health status, which may be used to account for differences among plans in the burden of illness. Furthermore, each insurer requests different pieces of information on enrollees resulting in a lack of uniformity across different enrollment files. Another problem with enrollment files is that they are based on insurance status, so anyone who resides in a community and who is uninsured is not included in these files. Strategies for obtaining information on the uninsured will be somewhat different (e.g., surveys) depending on the purpose of the analysis.

Improving the Quality of Enrollment Data. Much can be done to make enrollment files more useful for evaluation and quality-monitoring purposes, as Table 5.10 illustrates. The most important changes include (1) greater uniformity across systems in the required set of information that is collected, (2) an expanded set of variables to capture information on individuals that is germane to health care utilization, costs, and outcomes, and (3) regular updating of files by all health plans. Because these files are generated by employers and government programs, the improvements would need to be instituted across the variety of entities that maintain these files.

The data enhancements identified in Table 5.10 are critical to accurately evaluate differences in utilization of services, expenditures, and health outcomes. Integrated health data systems should make the inclusion of these elements a high priority.

Clinical Data

Definition. The most common source of clinical data is medical records maintained by hospitals and physicians. Medical records contain information on a patient's medical history, primary complaints, presenting symptoms, physical examinations, clinical assessments and diagnoses, diagnostic test results, procedures performed, medications, response to treatment, the clinical course of the patient, discharge plans, and demographic factors such as age and gender.

Table 5.10

Potential Enhancements to Enrollment Data

Unique identifier for the enrolled person and all dependents. This is important for linking information across the health system (hospital, doctor's office, pharmacy, and laboratory) on individual patients. Social Security numbers are not adequate for this purpose.

Demographic information such as education, race/ethnicity, gender, income, and marital status. These data elements are important to capture, since they frequently explain variation in the use of services and in health expenditures. At present, there are legal restrictions against the reporting of race, which will need to be addressed if this data element is desired.

Employment information on wage rate, industry code, hours worked per week, occupational status, firm size, and average payroll of firm. Because of the strong link between the provision of insurance and employment for the majority of Americans below age 65, the addition of these data elements can inform policymakers about the relationship between employment, health status, and health care costs and utilization.

Plan information about the type of coverage offered to and chosen by individuals (e.g., HMO, PPO, IPA, or FFS), names and birth dates of all covered persons under the plan, relationship to the primary enrolled person, enrollment and disenrollment dates, and characteristics of the benefit package (e.g., cost-sharing requirements and benefits covered). These data elements are important for understanding individual decisions about enrollment in health plans, defining the actual insured population, and evaluating the use of services in a particular plan over a defined time period.

Health information, including the health and functional status of all health plan members. Health and functional status information can be used for a variety of purposes including risk adjustment and understanding whether adverse selection is occurring among certain health plans. These measures can also serve to indicate whether the population has unmet health needs in relation to their observed utilization of services.

Frequency of updating to ensure that the denominator for rate calculations is as accurate as possible. Quarterly enrollment updates should be a minimum standard and monthly updates a maximum standard.

The information contained in medical records documents what occurred from the clinician's perspective—that is, what problem the patient reported, what tests or drugs were ordered, and what treatment/preventive recommendations were made. All of this information is confidential and special permission is required to gain access to any of the data contained in the medical record.

Potential Uses of Clinical Data. Clinical data are used to study access problems, the appropriateness of procedure use, quality of care, and clinical outcomes. Table 5.11 provides some examples of the potential uses of clinical data. The footnotes provide references for studies that used clinical data to address the illustrative question.

Data Elements. The greatest strength of medical records for health services research is that they provide the detailed clinical data that is necessary for evaluating the quality of care, even though the data can vary widely. Table 5.12 lists the type of information frequently found in a patient's medical record.

Table 5.11

Illustrative Uses of Clinical Data

Cost and utilization studies
    Examine factors that explain differences in costs among hospitals[a]
    Compare how the utilization of specific procedures varies for persons with
        particular medical conditions[b]
    Study the underuse of services by examining variations in the use of diagnostic
        tests, for a particular health condition, by age, gender, insurance status, or
        race
    Evaluate whether the application of medical procedures varies by age, race, or
        gender for the same health condition[c,d]
    Assess the timeliness of follow-up on abnormal laboratory or diagnostic test
        results

Quality of care
    Examine hospital outcomes as an indicator of quality of care[e]
    Evaluate the appropriateness with which various surgical procedures are used[f]
    Assess adherence to clinical practice guidelines
    Examine the effect of quality improvement activities at hospitals[g]

Outcomes evaluation
    Examine how health outcomes (e.g., in-hospital mortality rates) vary as a
        function of the volume of surgeries performed[h]
    Evaluate the relationship between the process of care and in-hospital mortality[i]
    Identify risk factors for surgical outcomes[j]
    Perform technology assessments to identify which treatment works best under
        what types of conditions

SOURCES: [a]Iezzoni et al. (1990); [b]Kleinman et al. (1994); [c]Greenfield et al. (1987); [d]Ayanian and Epstein (1991); [e]Dubois et al. (1987); [f]Hilborne et al. (1993); [g]Hannan et al. (1994); [h]Hannan et al. (1991); [i]Kahn et al. (1990); [j]Hannan et al. (1992a).

Clinical data represent the most important source of information about the details of diagnosis and treatment, patient risk factors, and the clinical outcomes of care. Data on demographic characteristics (age and gender), comorbidities, and disease severity are examples of data obtained from medical records that are necessary for risk adjustment. These data are required to examine differences in patient outcomes resulting from treatment. Furthermore, information in the medical record can point to poor outcomes that result from treatment, such as complications resulting from surgery or iatrogenic events (Iezzoni et al., 1990).

Limitations in the Use of Clinical Data. Several issues related to clinical data affect their use. Each patient can have multiple medical records that are the result of care provided by different doctors and hospitals. A new medical record is established each time the patient seeks care from a different inpatient or outpatient provider, which implies that to understand fully the care a patient received for a medical condition you would need to obtain all of that patient's medical records. Medical records are different from the previously discussed

Table 5.12

Information Typically Contained in a Medical Record

Patient information
    Patient name (first, last, middle initial)
    Address (street, city, state, zip code)
    Gender
    Date of birth
    Race/ethnicity (often unreliable)

Medical information
    Reason for visit or admission
    Diagnoses
    Stability of condition, severity of diagnosis
    Medical history—description of the problem
    Medications prescribed
    Physical exam findings
    Laboratory results (e.g., blood test, urine tests)
    Diagnostic procedures and results (radiology and imaging tests, blood pressure)
    Treatments provided (medical, surgical)
    Outcomes of or response to treatment (patient better or worse)
    Dates of service
    Follow-up care/plans
    Complications (not always noted in the record)
    Discharge status
    Referrals to other providers

Provider information
    Physician name or initials
    Other provider name or initials

sources of data because they have no standard format or procedures for recording patient information. In most cases, medical records cannot be directly used for analytic purposes because of the lack of uniformity, the information is often handwritten, and they tend to exist in hard copy format only.

Medical records also do not contain a unique individual identifier for patients that is common across all health care facilities or delivery systems. Again, this prevents easy linking to other data sources for more complex analyses. Also, because there is no uniformity in what physicians are required to document in a patient's medical record, many of the items listed in Table 5.12 may or may not be found in the record, or may vary in terms of their description. These factors make uniform comparisons difficult. To illustrate this point, if two patients with a similar medical condition received different treatments, you might want to identify the set of factors that may have influenced different decisions about treatment (e.g., different severity of illness, clinical findings, or history of care). If the information is not documented in the medical record, you could not understand what led to different decisions about treatment.

Today, when detailed clinical information about a set of patients is required for a study, the data have to be manually abstracted from medical records in a retrospective fashion (i.e., after care has been delivered). From the abstraction forms, researchers construct data elements or variables. Because most hospitals and medical offices currently maintain these records only on paper and since the entries are typically handwritten, the abstraction process is very costly and time-consuming. The information recorded in the file is also highly variable, adding a further complication to interpreting the information.

In addition, users need to be aware that medical record information reflects both the subjective evaluation of the provider and objective results from clinical tests. Before drawing conclusions about observed differences in outcomes, it is necessary to take account of the fact that physicians may differ among themselves on the diagnosis and the recommended course of treatment for the same patient. Additionally, doctors may forget to record information in the clinical record (e.g., prescription drugs or other treatment provided during a telephone consultation). Analysts should consider the possible reasons that information necessary to answer policy questions may not be in the clinical record and how that affects the ability to draw conclusions.

Improving the Quality of Clinical Data. Medical records can be made more useful for clinicians and for studies of the health care delivery system. In response to efficiency and quality improvement demands, providers are moving toward computerized entry of clinical data at the time of service, which will greatly improve the timeliness and accessibility of clinical data for a variety of purposes. Prospective collection of clinical information will also permit the expansion of the data elements that can be obtained (e.g., greater information related to treatment and outcomes for patients with chronic illnesses) and thus can improve our understanding of how the health system performs. Chapter Seven provides a more thorough discussion of recommended changes to the collection of clinical data that will improve the accessibility and utility of this data source for analysis.

Prospective ("real-time") entry of information will

- Facilitate the timeliness of data availability;

- Provide opportunities to prompt clinicians for more data on certain types of conditions or patient factors that may relate to treatment outcomes;

- Promote greater uniformity in the information that is used to evaluate clinical performance; and

- Prompt physicians to include information in the medical record that might otherwise be omitted.

As Chapter Seven describes, high-quality clinical data should capture certain key items such as a patient's age, gender, race/ethnicity, complications of care, comorbid conditions, procedures performed, the dates when procedures occurred, and the patient's discharge status.

Survey Data

Definition and Function of Surveys. A survey is a tool for collecting information from individuals (e.g., patients and physicians) and organizations (e.g., hospitals and insurers). Survey data are most often used to study special issues or populations that are not captured in the data systems previously described in this chapter. Because administrative, enrollment, and clinical data do not contain much information that is collected directly from individuals, surveys of health plan enrollees or patients can generate person-level information on such issues as patient satisfaction with care, functional and health status, quality of life, health habits, and the individual's usual source of care. Surveys of providers can enhance understanding of the type of services provided, hours of operation, and the type of patients seen. Surveys are conducted at all levels by a variety of groups, such as health plans, business coalitions, employers, provider associations, consumer advocacy groups, and local, state, and federal governments. Surveys can be conducted annually (e.g., Current Population Survey), continuously (e.g., National Health Interview Survey), periodically (e.g., National Medical Expenditure Survey), or one-time only (e.g., National Survey of Worksite Health Promotion).

Potential Uses of Survey Data. Table 5.13 lists some examples of how survey data can be used. The footnotes refer the reader to studies that illustrate uses.

Each survey varies in terms of the data elements it collects; therefore, unlike the previously described data sources, there is no standard set of data elements. Analysts using surveys conducted by someone else are advised to obtain the documentation pertaining to a given survey of interest, which should contain the sampling method used, a copy of the survey as fielded, and names and definitions of data elements. Variable lists can be easily misinterpreted, so examination of the documentation is critical. Information about the field experience is also important, such as response rates.

Sources of Survey Data. Survey data currently are available at a variety of levels, ranging from national surveys of health care costs and utilization to individual health plan surveys of access to services and patient satisfaction. A large number of surveys are sponsored by state public health departments and federal agencies, such as the U.S. Department of Health and Human Services (e.g., Agency for Health Care Policy and Research [www.ahcpr.gov], National Center for Health Statistics [www.cdc.gov/nchswww], Centers for Disease Control and

Table 5.13

Illustrative Uses of Survey Data

Health and functional status
Quantify the proportion of the population with limited functional status due to chronic health conditions
Assess the relationship between health status and use of health care services[a,b]
Determine how a particular treatment affects functional health status

Cost and utilization studies
Examine differences in the use of health services by insured and uninsured persons[a,b,c]
Identify the usual source of care for different groups of individuals[b,d]
Assess what proportion of the population receives preventive services[e]
Examine the effects of market competition in reducing hospital costs[f]
Explore predictors of out-of-plan utilization
Identify risk factors associated with underuse of preventive services[g]

Consumer satisfaction
Evaluate enrollee satisfaction with access to care and the care they have received[h]
Assess whether facilities are conveniently located to consumers and whether the hours of operation meet the needs of consumers[e]

Cost studies
Explore how personal expenditures on health care vary by type of health insurance plan[i]
Predict total expenditures for individuals at different stages of a disease (e.g., AIDS and cancer)

Outcomes evaluation
Evaluate functional outcomes among those enrolled in different health plans or under treatment by providers with different specialty training
Evaluate the relationship between satisfaction with care and functional outcomes

SOURCES: [a]Freeman et al. (1987); [b]Davis and Rowland (1983); [c]Trevino et al. (1991); [d]Baker et al. (1994); [e]Andersen et al. (1986); [f]Zwanziger et al. (1994); [g]Bates et al. (1994); [h]The Robert Wood Johnson Foundation (1987); [i]Vistnes (1992).

Prevention [www.cdc.gov]), the Department of Veterans Affairs (www.va.gov), and the Department of Defense (TRICARE health program for military dependents [www.ha.osd.mil/]). Additionally, other nonhealth-related government agencies collect health-related information, such as the Department of Labor's ongoing Current Population Survey (CPS) series (www.bls.census.gov/cps), which collects information on insurance coverage, and the Department of Agriculture's Survey of Food Intakes (www.usda.gov), which tracks nutritional information. Table 5.14 lists some important health-related surveys that may be useful for analytic purposes. The list is by no means exhaustive but is illustrative of the types of survey data potentially available to health analysts.

In addition to government-sponsored surveys, private sector organizations also conduct surveys. Examples include surveys sponsored by the National Committee for Quality Assurance, the Health Insurance Association of America, the American Medical Association, the Employee Benefits Research Institute,

Table 5.14

Sample Listing of Health and Demographic Survey Data

Survey Name	Sponsor Agency or Organization	Sample Size	Frequency	State Data Available	Web Address
Adult Use of Tobacco Survey	Centers for Disease Control and Prevention	12,000	Periodic	No	stats.bls.gov/oshhome.htm
Annual Survey of Occupational Injuries and Illnesses	U.S. Department of Labor, Bureau of Labor Statistics	290,000	Annual	Yes	www.arfsys.com
Area Resource File	Health Resources and Services Administration (HRSA), Bureau of Health Professionals	Compilation of data bases	Continuous	Yes	
Behavioral Risk Factor Surveillance System	Centers for Disease Control and Prevention	1,700	Continuous	Yes	www.cdc.gov/nccdphp/brfss
Census of the United States	U.S. Department of Commerce, Census Bureau	U.S. population	Every 10 years	Yes	www.census.gov
CPS	U.S. Department of Commerce, Census Bureau, and Bureau of Labor Statistics	> 50,000	Monthly	Yes	www.bls.census.gov/cps
Fatality Analysis Reporting System	National Highway Traffic Safety Administration	Total motor vehicle fatalities	Continuous	Yes	www.nhtsa.dot.gov/people/ncsa/fars.html
High School Senior Survey (Monitoring the Future)	National Institute on Drug Abuse, University of Michigan	16,000–19,000	Annual	No	www.isr.umich.edu/src/mtf
National Death Index	Centers for Disease Control and Prevention	All deaths	Continuous	Yes	www.cdc.gov/nchswww/about/otheract/ndi/ndi.htm
National Household Survey of Drug Abuse	Substance Abuse and Mental Health Services Administration	8,000	Periodic	No	www.samhsa.gov/oas/nhsda/nhsdafls.htm
National Survey of Worksite Health Promotion Activities	Department of Health and Human Services, Office of Disease Prevention and Health Promotion	1,400 worksites	One time	No	www.ntis.gov

Table 5.14 (continued)

Survey Name	Sponsor Agency or Organization	Sample Size	Frequency	State Data Available	Web Address
Hispanic Health and Nutrition Examination Survey (HHANES)	National Center for Health Statistics (NCHS)	12,000	One time	No	www.cdc.gov/nchswww/products/catalogs/subject/hhanes/hhanes.htm
National Ambulatory Medical Care Survey (NAMCS)	NCHS	Varies by survey	Annual	In some cases	www.cdc.gov/nchswww/products/catalogs/subject/namcs/namcs.htm
National Health Interview Survey (NHIS)	NCHS	50,000–130,000	Continuous	No	www.cdc.gov/nchswww/products/catalogs/subject/nhis/nhis.htm
National Health and Nutrition Examination Survey (NHANES)	NCHS	21,000	Periodic	No	www.cdc.gov/nchswww/about/major/nhanes/nhanes.htm
National Hospital Discharge Survey	NCHS	250,000 medical records	Continuous	No	www.cdc.gov/nchswww/about/major/nhcs/nhcs.htm
Medical Expenditure Panel Survey (MEPS)	Agency for Health Care Policy and Research (AHCPR)	24,000	Periodic	No	www.meps.ahcpr.gov
National Nursing Home Survey	NCHS	1,000/5,200 nursing homes, current residents	Periodic	No	www.cdc.gov/nchswww/about/major/nhcs/nhcs.htm
National Survey of Family Growth	NCHS	8,500	Periodic	No	www.cdc.gov/nchswww/about/major/nsfg/nsfg.htm

SOURCE: Adapted from U.S. Public Health Service (1990).

the Blue Cross/Blue Shield Association of America, the American Hospital Association, the American Association of Health Plans, organizations that are consultants to or represent groups of employers (e.g., Foster Higgins and the Chamber of Commerce), and national and regional business coalitions on health (e.g., Washington Business Group on Health and Pacific Business Group on Health). These surveys typically focus on issues that are important to members or constituencies served by these organizations and therefore cover a wide range of subjects, such as the number of uninsured, the number of providers of different specialties and their distribution across the state or nation, the amount of care that is uncompensated, and member satisfaction with a health plan or medical group. Rules on access to these data vary, but most of the data from surveys listed in Table 5.14 are available at some level of aggregation for research purposes.

Many questions require that new surveys be fielded to augment information contained in other existing data sources. Because of the complexity of this topic, we encourage those who want to learn more about surveys to obtain a book on survey design and to consult an expert (e.g., a statistician or psychometrician). There are numerous books on survey design to choose from, but we recommend Weisberg and Bowen (1977) and Moser and Kalton (1971). Chapter Eight of this book provides more information about how to design and conduct surveys and a brief description of some of the key features of surveys.

Limitations in the Use of Surveys. Surveys can provide useful information, but health data users should be aware of several issues related to their use:

* **Surveys can be costly to perform and should be performed only when an important need arises.** Often surveys are conducted to collect data that are not available through existing data sources.

* **The majority of surveys are designed as cross-sectional studies.** As a result, they allow you to evaluate only what is occurring at a given point in time as opposed to being able to examine the behavior or event over time. Cross-sectional data can produce results that vary significantly from surveys that capture behavior over a longer period of time. For example, 37 million Americans were estimated to be uninsured at a given point in time in 1992, whereas data drawn over the course of the year produced an estimate of 58 million people who were uninsured at some point during 1992 (Swartz, 1994).

* **The results derived from a survey may be biased for various reasons.** For example, the sample drawn from the population may not be representative or the survey may suffer from low response rates or poor recall on the part of respondents. If respondents differ from nonrespondents in important

ways, then the results of the survey are not likely to be accurate for drawing conclusions. Or, if individuals incorrectly recall what services they received, the conclusions may misrepresent what actually occurred. Such factors will influence the validity and reliability of the information for analytic purposes.

- **Surveys do not contain linking variables as a general rule.** It may not be possible to combine survey information with other information on the respondent. Removing linkage variables is often done to maintain the confidentiality of respondents. Unique identifiers (e.g., Social Security number, Medicaid number, or private insurance plan number) as well as other nonunique identifiers that can be used for linking purposes, such as name, address, zip code, or state, are usually removed from the data file before making it available for use by the public.

- **There can be significant delays in the release of the data after the survey is done.** Such delays affect the timeliness of the information.

Other Data Sources

Types of Data That Are Available. A host of other data sources are available from state and federal governments as well as private sources. These sources serve various functions and may augment administrative, clinical, or survey data for conducting analyses. Several of the most important data sources include

- Birth certificate files;
- Death certificate files;
- Birth defects registry;
- Disease registries (e.g., cancer and end stage renal disease);
- Provider files; and
- Facility files.

These data files are very useful for studying the health system. For example, birth and death certificate files can be used to track health outcomes; disease registries can facilitate monitoring changes in the incidence of diseases over time. Provider files can also be used to supplement other data sources to determine the set of providers who are practicing in a given geographic area, their specialty, and the type of reimbursement they accept (e.g., Medicaid provider). These data files have the unique advantage of providing complete listings or a census of the events or providers.

Limitations of Other Data Sources. Once again, the most important issue related to their use in combination with other data sources is the ability to link
records at the level of the patient or provider. As currently designed, these data
sources do not contain unique patient or provider identifiers that are commonly applied across data systems. An example will help illustrate this point.
Table 5.15 lists the data elements that are available from the National Center for
Health Statistics on the public use maternal and infant health data files
(www.cdc.gov/nchswww/about/major/nimhs/abnimhs.htm). The files do not
contain the date of birth for the infant, mother, or father or the birth certificate
number. These data elements may be obtained from state vital statistics offices
for research purposes if approved under the state's review process. The data elements that are available and will be released vary from state to state and must
be shown to be necessary for the analytic study.

One use of natality data is to understand the factors that contribute to poor infant outcomes, such as low birthweight. To link natality data to the mother's
hospitalization or prenatal care data (medical records and administrative data),
you would need to match the records using a nonunique identifier, such as
mother's name or the infant's date of birth. Because these linkage variables are
not unique to each person, you are bound to get some duplicate matches. You
could also fail to find a match in cases where the mother's name on the birth
certificate is slightly different from that on the administrative record (e.g., mis-
spelled on one record). You could also fail to match the records in cases where
the baby's last name is different from the mother's last name (e.g., the infant
uses the father's surname). The next section illustrates the process by which
linking occurs without a unique identifier.

PROBLEMS AND POTENTIAL SOLUTIONS TO IMPROVE THE UTILITY OF HEALTH DATA SYSTEMS

The previous section on data sources highlighted a number of concerns that
apply to all of the data sources that might be included in an integrated data system. The issues are important because they affect the ability of the analyst to
gain the maximum value from the health information that is available. Four
overarching issues must be addressed for integrated data systems to evolve into
maximally useful information systems. The issues apply to administrative, enrollment, clinical, and other (supplemental) data sources of information.

Lack of Unique Identifiers for Linking Purposes

Unique identifiers for patients, providers, and facilities do not exist in the current data environment. For example, each insurer, including Medicare and
Medicaid, has a different system for identifying enrollees and providers of care.

Table 5.15

Data Elements—Public Use Natality Data Files (1989–1995)

Data year
Residence of mother[a]
State[b]
County[b,c]
City[c]
Population size
Standard metropolitan statistical area[b,c]
Metropolitan and nonmetropolitan counties
Abnormal conditions of the newborn[d]
Age of father (single years, 10 and over)
Age of mother (single years, 10–49)
Apgar scores, 1 and 5 minutes[d]
Alcohol use[d]
Attendant at birth
Birth weight (in grams)
Complications of labor or delivery[d]
Congenital anomalies[d]
Day of week of birth
Education of mother and father[d] (single years, 0–17)
Gestation period (single weeks, 17–47)
Hispanic origin of mother and father[d]
Marital status[e]
Medical risk factors[d]
Method of delivery[d]
Nativity of mother
Obstetric procedures[d]
Place of birth (state[b] and county[b,c])
Place of delivery
Plurality
Pregnancy history
   Born alive, now living
   Born alive, now dead
   Interval since last live birth (in months)
   Live-birth order
   Month/year of last live birth
   Total-birth order
Prenatal care
   Adequacy of care (Kessner Index)
   Month of pregnancy care began
   Number of prenatal visits
Race of child (9 categories)
Race of father (10 categories)
Race of mother (9 categories)
Sex of child
Tobacco use[d]
Weight gain during pregnancy[d] (single pounds, 0–99)

SOURCE: CDC/NCHS (1998). Now called the National Maternal and Infant Health Survey

[a]The place of residence for mothers who were nonresidents of the United States has been coded to the country of residence.

[b]Includes FIPS codes as well as NCHS codes.

[c]Includes data for areas with a population of 100,000 persons or more.

[d]Applicable only for those states having information on the certificate.

[e]Data for states without the item have been inferred from other items on the certificate.

Individuals are identified on birth and death certificates with yet another identifier, and providers frequently have their own system for identifying patients
on medical records. Thus, any attempt to track the course of care for a given
patient in the system—by linking enrollment, administrative, and clinical
data—becomes difficult, if not impossible.

It is very important to be able to link data on individuals across settings of care
and across practitioners. Linking information by way of unique identifiers is
necessary to track individuals through the system and over time, so that their
full utilization and cost experience can be captured. Unique identifiers can facilitate the examination of practice patterns and the performance of hospitals,
physicians, and other medical providers over time and across the various systems of insurance.

Linking records from existing data files to form a new data file expands the
power of the information beyond that of the data contained in each separate
file (the principal goal of integrated data systems). Linking data from a variety
of sources can enable decisionmakers to obtain analyses that would otherwise
be impossible or prohibitively expensive. Almost any evaluation of health system performance requires linking one or more data files. Several examples illustrate this point:

- One ongoing concern about the Prospective Payment System of reimbursement is that hospitals have a financial incentive to discharge patients
  prematurely. To evaluate this concern, you would need information on (1)
  posthospital mortality (requires linking to death certificate data), (2) repeat
  admissions to hospitals including different hospitals (requires the ability to
  track patients across multiple hospitals), and (3) health status at admission
  to postacute care facilities (requires linking the same patient across different care facilities).

- To analyze the outcomes of hospital treatment for a heart attack, you would
  want to link death certificate and hospital readmission data to the patient's
  original encounter and clinical data to see what happened to the patient
  after being discharged from the hospital. Furthermore, data on the
  functional status of the patient could be linked from patient surveys.
  Patient and facility identifiers on each file are required to do this analysis.

- To compare outcomes of different hospitals, you need to be able to account
  for differences among admitted patients in their relative levels of illness at
  admission. One hospital may have a higher mortality rate than another
  hospital simply because it treats more terminally ill patients. The data
  sources might include medical record (prior treatment and clinical status at
  admission), administrative data (number of prior hospitalizations), or sur-

vey results (health status). A unique patient identifier is required to link these records.

- If you were studying birth outcomes, you would like to have information on each of the potential factors that contributed to the birth outcome, including (1) maternal and paternal health history, (2) quality of prenatal care, (3) labor and delivery, and (4) postdelivery care. These pieces of information are contained in different files (e.g., mother's prenatal care records, hospital medical record, and birth and death certificates). Linking these data sources requires having the same identifier for the mother on each file.

The best linking variable is one that is unique and permanent for each individual and provider, maintains individual privacy, and allows for verification. An undesirable linking variable is one that can be reassigned to different individuals over time, as occurs today with Medicaid identifiers in some states. The Medicare program has a better system for uniquely identifying Medicare beneficiaries, although there are problems with this system as well. Medicare uses the individual's Social Security number (followed by the letter A for the beneficiary and B for the spouse) as the Medicare claim identifier, which simplifies the linking process. Undoubtedly, the large number of studies performed on the Medicare population are, in part, attributable to the ease with which enrollment, encounter, and other data sources can be linked by Social Security number for Medicare beneficiaries.

The Institute of Medicine's Committee on Regional Health Data Networks raised a number of issues related to the establishment and use of a common identifier (Donaldson and Lohr, 1994). Although the Social Security number (SSN) has been considered as a potential candidate for a national health identifier, a number of problems with this widely used identifier were noted. Some of the major concerns include high potential for error (intentional and unintentional); some SSNs may be used by multiple persons, and there are no legal protections associated with the SSN, such as being deemed a confidential data element. Furthermore, because the SSN is widely used, its application to health data files raises concerns about the ease with which links could be made to other sensitive information on patients or providers. These security and privacy issues reduce the willingness to use the SSN as a unique identifier.

By establishing and using a common set of unique patient and provider identifiers across all health care data files, health data systems can provide a powerful analytic resource. Table 5.16 lists key data files and the data elements in these files that would require unique identifiers.

We recommend that data system managers consider the following actions to address these problems:

Table 5.16

Data Sources and Required Identifiers

Data Sources	Required Identifiers
Hospital discharge or claims files	Patient, hospital, physician, newborn, payor
Outpatient claims or encounter data	Patient, physician, payor
Drug claims	Patient, prescribing physician, payor
Death certificates	Individual
Fetal death certificate	Mother
Birth certificate	Infant, mother
Birth defects registry	Child, mother
Disease registry	Individual
Provider files	Facility
Physician files	Physician, group (if applicable)
Hospital financial data	Facility
Enrollment	Employer, government program

- Establish a unique identifier for each patient, health care provider, and health plan/payor to serve as a linking variable;

- Evaluate opportunities to make the number consistent with federal coding schemes, such as using the Medicare facility ID to ensure wider ability to link data;

- Evaluate privacy issues associated with the use of a unique identifier; establish procedures for who will have access to identifying information and under what conditions; and

- Design a system to issue and monitor the use of unique identifiers.

Varying Levels of Data Quality

As mentioned above, accurate coding of diagnoses and procedures varies widely. Furthermore, there is no consistency in what providers note in the medical record. If information does not appear in the record, the analyst is left with the possibility that either an intervention that did occur was omitted from the record or that the treatment did not in fact occur. The analyst has no way of determining the right answer, which limits the ability to draw conclusions. High-quality and complete data are the hallmarks of data files that will permit extraction of useful information.

Data system managers must ensure that quality-control systems are designed and in place to monitor the completeness and accuracy of data that feed into the system. Incentives—such as tying reimbursement to coding—can serve to promote better coding practices. The implementation of the Prospective Payment System was effective in getting hospitals to provide complete diagnosis and procedure codes, since reimbursement levels were tied to coding.

Because poor-quality data are a serious impediment to being able to study a problem, efforts to improve data systems should devote resources to ensuring that data are entered correctly and completely. New York State created an incentive for better coding of comorbid conditions by routinely publishing mortality data at the hospital and physician level (New York State Department of Health, 1992). The data are risk-adjusted to ensure that hospitals are compared fairly and providers have improved the coding of items that are used to adjust for differences in risk that may influence the outcome (e.g., age, gender, and comorbid conditions). Publishing malpractice rates of providers is another incentive that can improve the coding practices of providers. As is evident from this discussion, financial incentives can be very powerful in a competitive delivery system. Methods that could be used to improve data quality include

- Establish operational definitions for assigning diagnosis and procedure codes;

- Disseminate coding guidelines to providers and payors;

- Require full coding (all five digits) of diagnosis codes to distinguish differences in severity of illness/condition;

- Conduct periodic audits to assess accuracy of coding in encounter data and compare against clinical data;

- Provide financial incentives to encourage complete and accurate coding; and

- Begin the process of moving toward a clinical data system; prospective entry of data will prompt providers for important clinical information to adjust for differences in risks and build in systems to ensure greater accuracy and uniformity of coding.

Nonuniformity of Data Elements Across Different Data Systems

Because each insurer uses different coding systems and collects different variables, health plan or systemwide comparisons are difficult to make. Furthermore, in the case of enrollment files, insurers differ in how often they update this information. The specific data elements captured in today's clinical data files (medical records) vary widely and there is no uniformity in how events are described or recorded. Because of the need to compare patients, providers, and health plans, data system managers should agree on a basic, uniform set of data elements across different administrative, enrollment, and medical claims systems. Each insurer would collect the same demographic, cost, and health system data elements using a standard set of codes and definitions. Analysts could then match, one-for-one, data elements across different insurers to examine how costs and utilization of services vary as a function of plan characteristics or the characteristics of the enrolled population. Standardization will dramatically enhance the ability of analysts to provide answers to more complex and policy-relevant questions by enabling uniform comparisons. It will also reduce the cost associated with collecting, linking, and analyzing information. Steps to improve the uniformity of data elements across data systems include

- Identify a core set of data elements that must be collected by all payors and providers of care;

- Establish common definitions and coding conventions for core data elements;

- Redesign data collection tools to ensure uniformity; and

- Provide financial incentives to ensure the use of uniform coding on core data elements.

Enhancements to the Existing Set of Data Elements

As the preceding discussion has demonstrated, existing data files do not always contain important pieces of information required to conduct even the most simple analyses. The priorities we have identified for making enhancements to these data sources are summarized below.

- Review existing data forms to determine what is collected and what important elements are missing (e.g., health status);

- Build consensus among policymakers, payors, providers, and consumers on the important data elements that should be added; and

- Revise forms/collection tools to include missing items.

Chapter Six

GENERAL ANALYSIS ISSUES

by Elizabeth A. McGlynn, Sally C. Morton, and Cheryl Damberg

Analysis is the art of transforming data into information that can be used for decisionmaking. This chapter explores the basic steps of analysis:

- Defining the question to be answered;

- Designing the study;

- Identifying the data source;

- Constructing an analytic data set;

- Using various analytic techniques to arrive at possible answers to the question; and

- Interpreting the results of the analysis.

This chapter highlights issues that consumers of research should be aware of when requesting analyses of data and when examining the results presented by those who have done analyses. The chapter is not intended as a textbook introduction to analysis—it will not answer at a technical level questions about how to apply a variety of analytic and statistical techniques. However, it will facilitate an examination of analytic techniques used by others. Our discussion is aimed at readers who have taken an introductory statistics course.

To make this chapter more concrete and meaningful to the reader, we will use an illustration that carries through many different sections of the chapter. We have selected the area of childhood immunizations because it illustrates a broad range of questions that might be analyzed using the information contained in health data bases. Childhood immunizations raise questions regarding access to care, cost of services, and quality of care. One can obtain information about the proportion of the population that is immunized and their characteristics from a variety of sources including administrative, clinical, and survey data. Childhood immunization rates have been used to evaluate the performance of managed care plans and represent one of the nation's public health goals for the year 2000 (U.S. Public Health Service, 1990).

FORMULATING THE QUESTION

Analysis begins with formulating a question. The key is to formulate a question that can be answered; the more specific the question, the easier it will be to develop an answer to that question. For example, the following question might be a reasonable one to ask, but is so broad that it is difficult to answer directly: *What proportion of people in the state receive needed preventive services?*

To answer this question, you would need to

- Make a list of what services constitute "needed" preventive services;

- Determine who is the target population for each of those services;

- Decide how frequently the services should be received;

- Calculate separate rates for each service (the proportion of the target population receiving the service); and

- Decide how to average the individual rates to come up with an overall assessment that would answer the question as posed.

The issues around obtaining each type of preventive service—immunizations, mammography, or blood pressure screening—vary and the solutions to problems involving each type are likely to be different. Consequently, an overall assessment of preventive service use might not provide useful information for decisionmaking. Thus, a necessary step is to narrow the question to something you can more easily answer. For example: *During calendar year 1998, what proportion of children under age two were up-to-date on their immunizations?*

This question is an improvement over the previous question because it

- Provides a time frame (calendar year 1998);

- Specifies a target population (children under age two);

- Has an explicit performance indicator (up-to-date); and

- Identifies a single type of preventive service (childhood immunizations).

This question could be further specified by limiting the evaluation to a geographic area (e.g., in a single state or community) or to selected subgroups (e.g., by race/ethnicity, age, income, type of vaccine, or type of health insurance).

To arrive at a question that is sufficiently specific to be answered typically requires an iterative process. As you develop a question, you should consider:

- **Who is the potential audience for the answer?** Identifying the audience for the study will help you refine the question further. For example, an employer might be interested in knowing how well each of the health plans with which it contracts are doing in immunizing children. Does the employer care only about children of its employees or are overall health plan rates acceptable? Is it useful to compare the rates experienced by employees' children with those of other children enrolled in the health plan? Are there other comparisons that would be useful in interpreting whether health plans are doing a good or bad job? If a state health department is asking the question, the identification of the target population—that is, the population to whom the answer applies—might be quite different (e.g., uninsured and insured children).

- **Why is the question important to answer?** In general, it is useful to focus on answering questions that provide information for action. For example, questions that evaluate the quality of health care delivery might lead to *improvements in quality;* questions that compare the costs of delivering certain services among different organizations might help identify the most *efficient practices* and eventually lead to *cost reductions;* questions that examine whether different groups in the population are experiencing problems in accessing certain health services might lead to programs that *improve access to needed services.*

- **How will the answer be used?** It is also important to think about what actions might be taken in response to having a question answered. You would like to obtain enough information in answering the question to determine potential courses of action that might be taken to improve the situation or to make a decision. For example, if a state discovers that only 75 percent of its children are being immunized, it might undertake a program to reach some portion of the remaining 25 percent who are not currently immunized. For the state to act effectively, it is important to know whether the 25 percent are equally distributed across the population or concentrated among certain subgroups (e.g., uninsured children, children with chronic diseases, or children living in rural areas). Because analyzing data can be expensive, it is worthwhile to spend some time thinking through the implications of the answer before doing the analysis so that a related series of questions can be addressed at one time.

In developing a study question, we recommend evaluating the question along the dimensions shown in Table 6.1. This process will help identify areas for refinement and clarify the intent of the analysis.

Table 6.1

Checklist for Evaluating the Analytic Question

Who is the target population?
What is the time frame for analysis?
What is the problem you are trying to address?
Are single or multiple issues/problems being addressed?
Are the concepts measurable?
Who is the audience for the answer?
How will the answer be used?

If multiple issues or problems are addressed in a question, it may be best to separate the issues into distinct questions. The objective is to make questions focused and to avoid trying to answer questions that are too broad or too complex.

DESIGNING THE STUDY

Once you have selected the question, the next step is to design the study. The nature of the question may influence the choice of study design.

The primary focus of this book is on studies that use existing sources of data. Analyses of such data are generally called secondary analyses. In such situations, the analyst cannot control or change the study design for data already collected. However, he or she must understand how the study design affects analysis and the inference it is possible to draw about the target population from the study data.   The analyst may in fact be able to choose between secondary data sets with different designs.

We now briefly review the key features of study designs, keeping in mind that terminology varies across scientific fields. A thorough discussion of design is beyond the scope of this volume, and the reader is referred to the large body of statistical and epidemiological literature available (e.g., Campbell and Stanley, 1963; Cook and Campbell, 1979; Freedman et al., 1991; Kish, 1987; and Mausner and Kramer, 1985).

The basic way to test the effectiveness of any intervention is comparison. For example, how does a patient who receives an intervention compare to a patient who has not received the intervention? The former is often called a member of the "treatment group" and the latter a member of the "control group." Intuitively, you might wish to ask if these two patients are the same in all respects other than having received the intervention or not? Comparison groups, that is, one or more treatment groups and a control group, are often the basis for scientific inquiry and the way they are formed and the way the effect of the intervention is measured on them depend on the study design chosen.

The analyst's first step is to determine if a control group is included in the study. If one is not, the study may not yield much useful information.

If the study does have a comparison group, is assignment to the treatment and control groups under the control of the investigator? If so, the study is a *controlled experiment.* If not, the study is an *observational study.*

Observational studies may have inherent biases because the participants may have self-selected into one comparison group or the other. For example, a study that compares the health outcomes of smokers and nonsmokers may be susceptible to bias. If such a study concludes that smokers are healthier than nonsmokers, this nonintuitive conclusion may result because sicker participants do not choose to smoke, or have quit smoking because of the additional morbidity associated with smoking. Thus, the poor health outcomes in the nonsmoking group may result because nonsmokers are not as healthy as smokers to begin with, not because this group's members do not smoke.

In some situations, for ethical or practical reasons, observational studies may be the only study design possible. For example, it would be unethical to attempt to study the effects of smoking on health by randomly assigning people to be smokers or nonsmokers.

A common type of observational study is a "cohort study" in which a particular population is followed over a period of time. The population may naturally assign itself to an intervention or not, and the outcomes associated with that intervention may be studied. When working with observational data, the analyst must be mindful of its drawbacks and potential inherent biases and perhaps account for the fundamental differences between the treatment and control groups via modeling, as discussed below. A detailed discussion of the inference possible from various designs, especially in terms of causation, are given in Campbell and Stanley (1963) and Cook and Campbell (1979).

If the study is a controlled experiment, the analyst should then determine if individuals' assignment to treatment and control groups was randomized or not. If the study is randomized, it is commonly known as a "randomized controlled trial," abbreviated RCT. Randomization to the comparison groups guards against bias by attempting to balance the groups in terms of all other factors besides the intervention so that the effect of the intervention may be clearly distinguished from the effect of other variables, commonly known as "potential confounding factors."

The method and implementation of the randomization may have certain characteristics. For example, a study that compares patients who receive a new drug to those who do not receive any drug may be a "double-blind placebo RCT." In this type of study, both the investigator and the patients are "blinded" to assignment so that none of the participants know which group they have been assigned to. The investigator simply knows the group membership as "belonging to group A," or "belonging to group B." Regardless of his or her assignment, the patient takes a drug according to the protocol. That drug may be the actual drug or a placebo, that is, it may look and taste just like the drug but is not a drug. Only after the study has concluded and the analysis has been performed is the group membership revealed. Blinding controls for bias, unconscious or otherwise, on the part of the investigator or patients.

In addition, randomization may be stratified. For example, patients within certain subgroups (grouped by gender, for example) may be randomized separately. Such stratified randomization ensures that the comparison groups have an approximately equal number of men and women in each group. A wide array of literature is available on the science of randomized controlled trials.

The pool of patients available for assignment may also be formed in a variety of ways. In the preceding example, the control group is formed concurrently, that is, patients from a particular cohort (for example, all patients who come to a particular clinic during a specific month) are randomized to the comparison groups. Control groups may also be formed historically. For example, if all patients currently in a hospital receive a particular treatment, the control group may be a historical one consisting of all patients who came to the hospital last year before the treatment was in use.

"Case-control studies" are ones in which each case, that is, a participant who had a particular outcome or disease, is matched to a control participant who did not have the outcome. These two groups of patients are then compared in terms of the pattern of services and treatments each received. This design differs from those discussed previously because the comparison groups are formed based on the outcome of interest rather than on who received the intervention and who did not. Such a design is commonly used when the outcome is rare, and the finding or identification of cases is a challenge. Historical control group studies and case-control studies are discussed in more detail in Mausner and Kramer (1985).

When a control group is impossible to form for some reason, a patient may serve as his or her "own control." Studies that fall into this category take a measurement before an intervention and a measurement after the intervention and then examine whether differences exist. These are sometimes called "pre-post" designs. Such studies are often used when cost limits the construction of a true control group. As described in Cook and Campbell (1979), this design is limited in terms of the inference that may be drawn from it.

When considering the design of a study, the analyst should also note the timing of the comparison group construction and the measurement. For cohort studies, "prospective cohorts" are defined and then followed over time. "Retrospective cohorts" are defined and then measured using historical data. Retrospective cohorts may be susceptible to bias because the historical measurements may not have been taken very accurately. In a prospective cohort, the study investigators can control the measurement process, making sure it is accurate and consistent. These designs are discussed in detail in Mausner and Kramer (1985).

Studies are also categorized according to whether they are "cross-sectional" or "longitudinal." In cross-sectional studies, both the group membership—i.e. whether the patient received the intervention—and the outcome are measured at a single point in time. In longitudinal studies, the group membership is usually measured before the outcome. Additionally, several outcome measurements may be taken over time so that the stability of the intervention may be evaluated—for example, does the effect dissipate? As discussed in Cook and Campbell (1979), longitudinal designs are stronger in terms of the inference that can be drawn.

Most information systems will be built around observational data, either from administrative or survey sources. Experimental data are rarely available for secondary analysis. This means that analysts must account for the inherent limitations of observational data in choosing the research question, conducting the analysis, and interpreting the results. These data may be useful for guiding policy decisions or formulating future research that uses stronger designs.

IDENTIFYING THE DATA SOURCE

Both the question and the study design contribute to identifying the data that are necessary to conduct the study. As described in Chapter Five, a variety of data sources are available in the health system. Some questions may be answered using a single source of data, whereas others require combining multiple sources of data. In some cases, such as the example of childhood immunizations, there may be more than one type of data that could be used to answer the question, such as survey and clinical data. The decision should be driven by determining what type of data are likely to produce the most accurate answer or contain the most complete information and by the relative cost of obtaining data from each potential source.

A common aid for matching questions with appropriate data sources is a catalogue of what information is available from different data sources. In Chapter Five, we listed common data elements found in various types of data (e.g., see Tables 5.3 and 5.4 for examples from inpatient and outpatient encounter forms). Table 6.2 shows what types of data might be useful for answering the above question about childhood immunizations. In this example, at least two

Table 6.2

**Determining Data Requirements: Childhood
Immunization Example**

Data Requirement	Data Type
Target population	
Children under age two	Enrollment
Other demographic characteristics	Enhanced enrollment
Timeframe	
Calendar year 1994	Administrative
	Clinical
	Survey
Topic	
Immunizations	Administrative
	Clinical
	Survey
Indicator (performance measure)	
Up-to-date	External standards
	(e.g., PHS, specialty society)

data sources are required to answer the question as posed. Enrollment data are needed to identify the target population who should receive the service, whereas information about who among the target population actually received immunizations could be obtained from administrative, clinical, or survey data—either singly or in combination. The performance indicator (up-to-date) could be determined by reference to existing standards of care either from the U.S. Public Health Service, which has made recommendations regarding the provision of preventive services, or similarly from an appropriate specialty society (e.g., the American Academy of Pediatrics). The question, as formulated, suggests an observational design.

Table 6.2 illustrates one approach to determining what data sources will be required. The approach identifies the individual elements of the question to be answered and, for each critical aspect of the question, considers what data source might contain the appropriate information. This process will help the analyst choose catalogues of data elements that should be examined to determine an optimal data strategy.[1]

Because multiple data sources are required to answer the question, it will be necessary to link information at the level of the individual across different data sources. For example, if you think about answering this question for a single health plan you would identify children in the appropriate age range using enrollment files from the health plan and then examine whether those children

---

[1]Data dictionaries represent one type of catalogue of data elements.

had received immunizations as recorded in administrative or clinical data sets or by surveying their parents. It is critical to make sure that the children you identify as being in the correct age range using the enrollment data are identical to those for whom you examine immunization rates using administrative, clinical, or survey data.[2] If the data sources contain information on different children, the rates are likely to vary with the data source and it may be difficult to determine the correct rate.

In this example, for two aspects of the question—time frame and topic—three possible data types could be used: administrative, clinical, or survey data. How do you choose a data source if there is more than one option? It is important to emphasize that there may not be one "correct" answer. Instead, we will describe a process to help you evaluate which data source is likely to be the best for your purposes. Because no data source is perfect, the process involves evaluating the strengths and weaknesses of your data options in the context of your analysis. In some cases, it may be helpful to compare the answers you would get from using one type of data rather than another. By doing so, you will test how sensitive your results are to the choice of data source. The process we illustrate in Table 6.3 is one that is designed to consider issues related to the quality and completeness of the potential data source.

Both administrative and clinical data sources share the problem that if the immunization was provided by an entity (i.e., health plan, clinic, or doctor) other than the one being evaluated, there may not be a record of the child having received the service. Survey data are more likely to capture the child's immunization experience across different service providers (e.g., health plan, county health department, or school clinic) but are affected by whether the parent remembers accurately which immunizations were given and on what date. For parents who maintain a formal record of this information, the responses may be quite accurate; if the response is based simply on what the parent recalls, it is subject to errors in recall that may bias the results (i.e., parents may report too many or the wrong dates). This is an example of response bias. The types of problems listed may not be completely avoidable (e.g., missing data), but it is important to evaluate the magnitude of these problems and to consider possible solutions. This is discussed in more detail in the section below on Initial Data Quality Checks.

Table 6.4 illustrates the kind of information for which each source of data is a good or poor source of information. In some cases, the information may not be available from a particular source. In other cases, there are clear advantages to one source of data over another.

---

[2]See Chapter Five for a discussion of linking data using unique identifiers.

Table 6.3

Evaluation of Data Quality and Completeness: Illustrative Examples

Data Type	Potential Problem	Category of Problem[a]
Adminis-trative	Will a claim exist for an immunization? In some organizations, this may be included as part of a well-child visit and not separately billed	Missing data Comparability[b]
	Consistency of coding practices (e.g., same use of CPT-4 codes)	Dissimilar data across different entities
	No claim if immunization not done by health plan	Missing data
	Date of immunization missing	Missing data
	Dependents or ages of dependents missing	Missing data
Clinical	No record if immunization not done by health plan	Missing data
	Record cannot be located	Missing data
	Date of immunization missing	Missing data
	Type of immunization not recorded	Missing data
Survey	Sample was drawn improperly	Selection bias
	Response rate less than 80 percent	Nonresponse bias
	Some questions not answered	Response bias
	Questions answered inaccurately	Measurement error

[a]The problems of missing data, measurement error, selection bias, and response bias are defined and discussed below.

[b]Comparability refers to whether or not the data are similarly collected so that comparisons can be made across different sources of data.

Table 6.4

Strengths and Weaknesses of Data Sources

Data Source	Good Information Available	Information Lacking/Limited
Administrative	Visit patterns Use of lab and diagnostic tests Prescriptions filled	Visit content Test results and follow-up Compliance with prescribed medication regimens
Clinical	Technical aspects of care Test results Inpatient processes of care	Interpersonal aspects of care Normal physical exam findings Outpatient processes of care
Survey	Symptoms Interpersonal aspects of care Care from all providers	Clinical findings Technical processes

There are no perfect choices in selecting data sources; each type involves making tradeoffs with respect to ease of use, accuracy, and content. Some of the major tradeoffs to consider are the following:

• Who is included in the data source and who is excluded?

• For what time period is the information available?

• How much will it cost to obtain information from each data source?

- How easy or difficult will it be to conduct analyses on each data source?

- How accurate will the results be from each data source?

Each choice will require different techniques to optimize the use of the data set to answer the question of interest. It is important to think ahead, however, about the likely set of problems that will be encountered. Understanding a data set's limitations will assist the analyst in designing optimal analytic strategies to minimize the effects of any data problems.

CONSTRUCTING AN ANALYSIS FILE

Having identified the sources of data to answer the question, the next step is to assemble data for analysis. This is generally referred to as constructing the analysis file. The purpose of this step is to reduce a large set of data to only that subset of data elements or observations needed for your particular analysis. It is generally most efficient to bring all of the necessary data together into a single file. Such analytic files can be constructed for the duration of the analysis and then either archived or destroyed once the project ends.

To construct an analysis file, several decisions must be made:

- Whether to restrict the file to the sample of people you are interested in studying and, if so, the criteria to use to restrict the sample;

- Which variables to include;

- How different data sources will be merged; and

- What initial data quality checks are required.

The objective at this point in the analysis is to get the data ready for analysis—to make the data set as error free as possible before beginning the initial steps in answering the question of interest. In this section, we will consider data that already exist (often called secondary data, meaning that the data were originally collected for a primary purpose other than the current one). For issues related to conducting surveys, see Chapter Eight.

Restricting the File to a Subset of Individuals

When working with large data sets, it is common practice to select a subset of individuals for analysis. This selection can be done by either restricting the analysis to all individuals for which the analysis is applicable, or by drawing a *probability sample* of those individuals for which the analysis is applicable, or both. A probability sample is a randomly drawn subset of individuals from a population in which each individual has a known probability of being sampled.

For the immunization example, we are interested only in children who are age two and younger and do not need information on any other individuals; thus, we will restrict the analysis file to all children age two and younger. As an example of a probability sample, most analyses done on Medicare claims data use just 5 percent of the entire population of claims submitted because analyzing a data set that contains information on millions of individuals would be expensive and time-consuming. A properly drawn probability sample will produce essentially the same results as analyzing the complete data set. To draw conclusions about the entire population from the sample, it is necessary to know, however, the probability with which any individual will be sampled.

If we want to represent the entire population of Medicare claims, we could take a simple random sample of 5 percent of the claims records. A simple random sample means that each claim has an equal sampling probability of 0.05 and each claim represents 20 claims in the population. Twenty is this individual's *sampling weight* in our analysis and is the inverse of the claim's probability of being sampled (1/0.05). Weights are used in combining information across the sample into estimates of population characteristics. For example, that claim's contribution to the estimated total number of hospitalizations experienced by all patients in the population is 20 times the number of hospitalizations recorded in that claim. If the elements in the population have different probabilities of being sampled, the sample is still a random sample although not a simple one, and the elements have different sampling weights. The sampling weights allow us to combine the information we gather from the sample so that we properly represent various components of the population. Statistical calculations discussed below can help determine how large the sample must be to confidently answer the questions of interest.

Choosing a method for obtaining subgroups (i.e., restricting to a certain subgroup of all individuals, drawing a sample, or some combination of these methods) depends on the questions being answered and the amount of data available. For many analyses, the starting point will be to identify characteristics of individuals on whom the analysis will be conducted (i.e., the target population). These characteristics might include age, geographic location, insurance status, time frame, and so on. If you are studying people with a particular disease, such as diabetes, the key subsetting variable will be one that identifies persons with the disease of interest. Once the group of persons with the characteristics of interest is identified, it may be desirable from a logistical viewpoint to further limit the number of persons in the analysis file by selecting a sample of eligible individuals. If a sample is drawn, the simple random sampling technique (i.e., all eligible individuals have an equal probability of being sampled), which is easily accomplished by a computer, is preferred because of greater simplicity in analysis. There are instances in which a different approach would be acceptable, but any deviation from simple random sampling should be adequately justified by a statistician.

In the childhood immunization example, we would begin by identifying all children under the age of two in the data set. Say, for example, there were one million persons in the state and 5 percent were in the target age group (N = 50,000). Then we might examine how the population of children are distributed by key variables as shown in Table 6.5.

Table 6.5, a frequency table showing the number of children in different population subgroups, represents one method for describing your data. One thing that becomes apparent in looking at these numbers is that there are very few American Indian, Eskimo, and Aleut children in the state, and there will probably be little statistical capacity to say anything about how their immunization rates differ from those of children in other ethnic or racial groups. This becomes even more problematic if you think about combining some of these variables. For example, suppose you were interested in *Hispanic* children in *rural* areas who were *uninsured*. You might estimate that 10 percent of the 4,750 Hispanic children also live in rural areas and are uninsured, which would produce a subsample size of 475 children who have these three characteristics. The estimated proportion of 10 percent may be derived from research literature or past experience with similar populations. A naive estimate from Table 6.5 would be 143 children (9.5 percent Hispanic x 25 percent rural x 12 percent uninsured = 0.285 percent of 50,000). This naive number underestimates the sample size as it assumes, for example, that the probability that a rural child is uninsured is the same as the probability that an urban child is uninsured. However, even if the naive estimate is the only one available, the exercise of estimating the likely number of persons who fall into each of the subgroups of interest, including combined subgroups, is instructive and recommended.

Table 6.5

Frequency Count of Children by Various Characteristics

Sample Characteristics	Frequency	Percent
Total number of children age two	50,000	100.0
White, not Hispanic	37,500	75.0
Black	5,900	11.8
Hispanic	4,750	9.5
American Indian, Eskimo, and Aleut	350	0.7
Asian/Pacific Islander	1,500	3.0
Urban	37,500	75.0
Rural	12,500	25.0
Insured, private	34,000	68.0
Insured, Medicaid	10,000	20.0
Uninsured	6,000	12.0

The sample size of 475 children is a small number of children to analyze and is one reason that many analyses use fairly broad groupings of characteristics (e.g., white or nonwhite). Precision and power analysis is a certain type of statistical analysis that can help you determine how large your sample should be for you to obtain useful estimates and to compare subgroups in a meaningful way. (This analysis will be discussed in more detail below.) After assessing a precision and power calculation, you may decide whether certain subgroup analyses will be feasible under the present sampling plan or whether you should oversample certain subgroups to increase your statistical power to detect a difference. In this example, you might take a random sample of 5 percent of the white ethnic group, and a 20 percent random sample from each of the other four ethnic groups. This stratified random sample would ensure that you could conduct useful subgroup analyses, which is one reason for deviating from simple random sampling.

Selecting Variables

In addition to selecting a subgroup of individuals for analysis, most questions will require only a small number of the variables drawn from the larger data set. The analysis file should contain only those variables that are required for the study. Variables can be classified as either

- **Dependent variables:** the outcome of interest or response that you want to understand (e.g., whether a child is immunized or not); or

- **Independent variables:** factors that influence or are related to the dependent variable (e.g., the child's ethnicity, whether the child lives in a rural or urban area, the child's health insurance status). Independent variables are sometimes called covariates.

You can identify the variables that will be required and the original data source from which those variables may be drawn. The example in Table 6.6 illustrates how you might select variables for the childhood immunization question.

In this example, three types of variables were selected from the various data sources:

1. **Individual characteristics:** Information on the characteristics of individuals was obtained primarily from enrollment data. The unique enrollee identifier and date of birth were obtained from each source so that data from different sources can be linked together. Often it is advisable to select more than one linking variable (e.g., name and date of birth), since the linking may occur in a stepwise fashion to reduce the possibility of mismatches; this is particularly true if a unique identifier is not available. The variables selected on

Table 6.6

Selecting Variables for the Analysis Data Set by the Potential Source of Data

Variable	Data Source			
	Enrollment	Administrative	Clinical	Survey[a]
Individual characteristics				
Enrollee identifier	x	x	x	x
Date of birth	x	x	x	x
Gender	x			
Race/ethnicity	x			
Household income	x			
Insurance status	x			
Geographic location	x			
Variables for immunization indicator (CPT-4 codes)				
DPT				
Date 1		x	x	x
Date 2		x	x	x
Date 3		x	x	x
Date 4		x	x	x
OPV				
Date 1		x	x	x
Date 2		x	x	x
Date 3		x	x	x
Measles				
Date 1		x	x	x
Mumps				
Date 1		x	x	x
Rubella				
Date 1		x	x	x
H influenza type B				
Date 1		x	x	x
Characteristics of the health system				
Miles to nearest facility				x
Hours of operation				x
Waiting time to visit				x
Fees				x
Pediatric visits per week				x
Broken appointment rates				x

[a]Survey data may not contain information on the same individuals that will be found in the other data sources. If unique or other nonunique (e.g., name and address) identifiers are not contained on the file, it may be difficult to link survey data to the other data sources. Chapter Five provides a more thorough discussion of this topic. The CPT-4 procedure codes are DPT (90701), oral polio virus (OPV) (90712, 90713), measles (90705, 90707, 90708), mumps (90704, 90707, 90709), rubella (90706, 90707, 90708) and H influenza type B (90737).

individuals will allow us to examine whether there are any differences in the rates at which children are immunized that are related to sociodemographic characteristics. These variables serve as independent variables in the analysis.

2. **Variables for immunization indicator:** In this example, information on the provision of each type of immunization is obtained to allow us to construct the pattern of service for each child. Since a child either received or did not receive an immunization, this variable is of a particular type and is referred to as an indicator or dummy variable (1 = yes; 0 = no). For this study, you can see that it is important to know for each type of immunization how many of the immunizations should be received between birth and age two. The schedule of immunizations for diphtheria, pertussis, and tetanus (DPT) requires a series of four shots before age two as compared to measles, mumps, and rubella (often given together and referred to as MMR), which requires only a single shot. We need to know the date that each of these shots was received to determine how old the child was when the shot was obtained. Immunization indicators serve as dependent variables in the analysis.

3. **Characteristics of the health system:** Information on the characteristics of the health system is obtained to understand whether aspects of service delivery either promote or inhibit timely immunization. This information could be found in data bases that maintain information at the facility level. What we would want to do in this case is to link information about different health plans to each individual who receives services at that plan: To obtain information on health plan characteristics, the linking variable is the health plan rather than the individual. Characteristics of the health system also serve as independent variables.

Thinking ahead about what information might explain differences in the question you are analyzing is important so that the analysis data set is complete. It is expensive to add variables to the analysis data set as a result of a second or third extraction process. On the other hand, you should be parsimonious in the selection of variables; the study question should be the principal determinant of variable selection.

Having catalogues of variables (e.g., data dictionaries) available on each data set that you can draw from will significantly facilitate constructing an analysis file. One reason is that the particular variable you may want to use might not be on the data base, so that you may need to select several variables to create a new variable (referred to as a derived variable) or use a variable that is similar to the desired variable that captures the idea of interest (referred to as a proxy variable). The catalogue will reduce the iterative process of placing a request for certain variables and then having to reconstruct the request based on information about the availability of data.

Merging Data from Different Sources

Because the analysis of immunization rates requires information from more than one source of data, we will have to merge the data sources to create a single record for each individual in the data set. Depending upon the analysis, the choice of a merging or linking variable may differ. If you are conducting analyses about individuals, then a unique individual identifier is the best choice for a merging variable. Such identifiers are not widely used today because of concerns about protecting an individual's right to privacy. If you are analyzing information about institutions (e.g., hospitals), then the identifier for the hospital, health insurance plan, or other institution may be the best merging variable. If unique identifiers are not available, merging data sources becomes substantially more difficult. The fallback option is to link records on other identifiers that are nonunique but that provide for relatively high rates of matching (e.g., name, date of service, or date of birth).

To illustrate the importance of having unique identifiers, we briefly summarize one method that was used to link vital statistics files with Medicaid claims data to examine the survival and health costs of very-low-birthweight infants (Bell et al., 1994). The study was conducted for the period 1980 through 1987, so several years of data had to be combined as well. Table 6.7 shows the list of potential linking variables for the two data sources.

Because the California vital statistics file and the Medicaid file use different codes to identify hospitals (i.e., there is not a unique identifier for hospitals in the state), hospital could not be used as a linking variable directly. In addition, because the study covered multiple years, the problem of hospitals changing names or locations, merging, and going out of business had to be dealt with in preparing the data for analysis. The steps required included

Table 6.7

Potential Linking Variables

Vital Statistics File	Medicaid File (Data Source)
Hospital ID or name	Hospital ID or name[a]
Last name of mother	
Last name of child	Last name of beneficiary[b]
First name of child	First name of beneficiary[b]
Age of mother in years	Birth date of mother and/or child[a,b]
Delivery date	Dates of hospital admission and discharge[a]
Zip code of mother[c]	Zip code of beneficiary

[a]Medicaid claims file.
[b]Medicaid enrollment file.
[c]Zip code was not on the vital statistics file in 1980–1981.

- Creating a cross-reference between hospital codes and hospital names and addresses;

- Standardizing data formats and abbreviations;

- Making an initial link by computer, using zip code and the first six characters of the hospital name and then zip code and the first 10 characters of the hospital address;

- Reviewing linked and unlinked hospitals with some links and making corrections by hand;

- Contacting hospitals directly to confirm name and location changes; and,

- Creating a final linking file.

This process creates a unique linkage. These steps could have been avoided if a unique identifier existed.

The next step was to link vital statistics and Medicaid records (information on particular individuals from each data source). This study attempted to develop an efficient procedure. The linking procedure that was developed addressed four issues:

- Requiring perfect agreement on all linking variables would result in a substantial number of matches being missed.

- Counting the number of agreements is an inefficient procedure. Not all matches provide equally strong evidence for linking. For example, mother's last name provides stronger evidence for a match than the mother's age in whole years because the probability of two names being the same is lower than the probability that two women would be the same age.

- Evidence on disagreement should be valued in relationship to the likelihood that the variable is coded correctly; disagreement on variables that are generally coded accurately (e.g., birthdate) provides stronger evidence of a mismatch than disagreement on variables that tend to be coded inaccurately (e.g., zip code).

- Even within a variable, some information may be more valuable than others. For example, linking an unusual name provides more information than linking a common name.

In developing the linking procedure, the authors were concerned principally with avoiding false positives (i.e., linking pairs of records that were not correct matches). The authors developed a scoring procedure that weighted all of the information on linking variables and then set a cutoff point that was likely to minimize the number of false positive matches without sacrificing too many potentially correct matches.

The authors' strategy required several steps and a manual review of some links at the final stage.

The key point is that without a unique identifier, linking data bases to explore common questions about the delivery and cost of health care can be time-consuming and expensive. Concerns about privacy are likely to limit the availability of unique identifiers. Thus, care must be taken in linking files and merging data sets, to prevent biases of unknown magnitude or direction being introduced into the conclusions.

Initial Data Quality Checks

Once the analysis data set is assembled, you should evaluate the quality of the data. There are several ways in which the quality of the data may be assessed:

- Check for common data problems;

- Address problems of missing data;

- Identify errors in measurement;

- Identify possible sources of bias;[3] and

- Select an approach to deal with bias.

These steps are discussed in more detail below.

Check for Common Data Problems. The first step in evaluating the quality of your data is often referred to as "cleaning" the data set. Two common types of data problems to look for are (1) out-of-range values and (2) lack of internal consistency.

Out-of-range values are numbers that are not reasonable values for the variable in question. For example, the gender variable will be coded with two values, such as 1 for males and 2 for females. If values other than 1 or 2 are found in the

---

[3]Any time we use a sample value to estimate a population value, such as using the average age of our sampled individuals to estimate the average age of the population, we need to be concerned about error in our estimate. Error in a sample estimate consists of two parts: (1) random sampling error and (2) bias. Random errors are not problematic, since they tend to offset each other when the measurements are averaged. Random error may be decreased by increasing the sample size. Bias, in contrast, is systematic and does not cancel out; it can make the conclusion you draw from your sample different from the true population result you are trying to estimate. Increasing the sample size does not decrease bias. Only changing the sampling technique or estimation procedure decreases bias. See Chapter Eight for a discussion of sampling techniques.

data set, this represents an out-of-range value. Another example of an out-of-range value is a birth date that results in ages that are either impossible (e.g., less than 0) or suggest that the person should not be included in the analysis (in the immunization example, older than age two).

How do you detect out-of-range values? You can begin by looking at the data in a number of different ways. A sample of one approach is shown in Table 6.8.

A couple of points need to be made about this example. First, for easy identification, many statistical software packages insert "." to designate missing values for a variable and to prevent the insertion of a numeric value that might inadvertently be analyzed (e.g., zero, 99). Zero is not used to indicate "missing" or

Table 6.8

Sample Frequency Table for Immunization Analysis

Variable Values	Frequency	Cumulative Frequency	Percent	Cumulative Percent
Gender				
. (missing)	500	500	1.0	1.0
1 (male)	24,300	24,800	49.6	50.6
2 (female)	25,000	49,800	50.0	99.6
9 (unknown)	200	50,000	0.4	100.0
Race/Ethnicity				
. (missing)	2,000	2,000	4.0	4.0
1 (white)	35,200	37,200	70.4	74.4
2 (black)	4,500	41,700	9.0	83.4
3 (Hispanic)	3,750	45,450	7.5	90.9
4 (American Indian/ Eskimo/Aleut)	200	45,650	0.4	91.3
5 (Asian)	1,300	46,950	2.6	93.9
9 (unknown)	2,000	48,950	4.0	97.9
11	200	49,150	0.4	98.3
13	500	49,650	1.0	99.3
15	350	50,000	0.7	100.0
Insurance status				
. (missing)	4,000	4,000	8.0	8.0
1 (private insurance)	29,200	33,200	58.4	66.4
2 (Medicaid)	8,500	41,700	17.0	83.4
3 (uninsured)	4,000	45,700	8.0	91.4
9 (unknown)	4,000	49,700	8.0	99.4
12	200	49,900	0.4	99.8
13	100	50,000	0.2	100.0
Geographic location				
. (missing)	2,500	2,500	5.0	5.0
1 (urban)	36,000	38,500	72.0	77.0
2 (rural)	10,000	48,500	20.0	97.0
9 (unknown)	1,000	49,500	2.0	99.0
19	500	50,000	1.0	100.0

"unknown" because it is a value with meaning; for example, zero visits to a doctor means something different from an unknown number of doctor visits. It is important to be aware of how your statistical computer software program handles missing data. For example, many programs drop observations with missing data from the analysis. In this example, it is easy to identify the extent to which data are missing for each variable. Second, many coding systems have an automatic data entry code for "unknown" values; we have used "9" in this example because this is a common coding convention.

Out-of-range values are those for which no pre-established category exists. In the example, for race/ethnicity, this includes codes 11, 13, and 15. For insurance status, the out-of-range values are 12 and 13, and for geographic location the out-of-range value is 19. A computer program can be written to review all variables to be used in the analysis and to flag values that are not acceptable. This process is essential when dealing with large data sets.

Internal consistency checks look at whether all the data for an individual appear to be feasible if examined together. For example, if the date of a vaccine is before a child was born this would be considered a consistency problem. The other type of consistency check is to compare information from different sources on the same question. For example, if we had information on the dates of immunizations from both encounter and clinical records, we could check to see if these two sources were in agreement about which immunizations were received and on what date. Table 6.9 shows a brief example of consistency checks.

The numbers under each variable name are the identifiers for each individual in the data file (0001–0005). In this example, the information about (1) birth date, (2) DPT date 1, and (3) DPT date 2 can be linked for a particular person. We can see that person 0001 was born on June 20, 1993, and received the first DPT vaccination on August 19, 1993, and the second vaccination on October 21, 1993. The information on birthdate could potentially come from each of the three data sources, whereas the information about immunizations will come from only the administrative and clinical data sets (for this example we are not considering the survey data file).

Two types of inconsistencies are illustrated in this example. The first is disagreement across data sources. Three of the individuals (0001, 0004, and 0005) have birthdates that agree across all sources. For person 0002, the enrollment and administrative data agree on the date of birth, but the clinical data set has a different date (although only four days off). For person 0003, the day and month are the same across all three sources, but the year is different in the administrative data. For person 0004, the dates of the first DPT shot in the administrative and clinical data sets differ by two months. The same problem occurs

Table 6.9

Sample Output for Consistency Checks
(inconsistent entries shaded)

Variable/ID	Enrollment	Data Source Administrative	Clinical
Date of birth			
0001	06-20-93	06-20-93	06-20-93
0002	08-19-94	08-19-94	08-15-94
0003	05-30-93	05-30-92	05-30-93
0004	03-10-93	03-10-93	03-10-93
0005	12-08-94	12-08-94	12-08-94
DPT date 1			
0001	—	08-19-93	08-19-93
0002	—	10-19-94	10-19-94
0003	—	08-05-92	08-05-92
0004	—	05-20-93	07-28-93
0005	—	02-15-95	06-30-94
DPT date 2			
0001	—	10-21-93	10-21-93
0002	—	12-20-94	12-18-94
0003	—	10-17-92	10-17-92
0004	—	07-28-93	09-30-93
0005	—	04-29-95	02-15-95

for the second DPT shot. This is a more subtle type of inconsistency to identify; what may have happened here is that the first DPT shot was not recorded in the clinical record and so the clinical data file counts the first recorded shot as the first shot—but in this case it is probably the child's second shot.

When the data across sources are inconsistent, you will have to develop a decision rule for choosing a single value for the variable.

For example, you could decide that the enrollment file is likely to be the most reliable source of information about basic demographics of individuals (e.g., date of birth) and you could select that as the primary source of information. You would prefer information from that source over all other sources if the variable is a demographic one. Another approach that could be used is, if two of the three sources agree, you could decide that the "majority rules."

The second type of inconsistency that is illustrated is events occurring out of sequence within a data source. For example, person 0003 shows a birthdate of May 30, 1993, on the clinical data set and a first DPT shot on August 5, 1992— before the person was born. For person 0005, the first shot occurs before the birth of the individual and the second shot occurs two months after birth. It is common practice to put events in chronological order and use that ordering to make variable assignments such as DPT date 1, DPT date 2. If, however, there is an error in the dates, this can introduce problems into the entire sequence of events. In the case of person 0005, DPT shot 1 is probably two months after birth (February 15, 1995; consistent with encounter data and second clinical date). DPT shot 2 is probably April 29, 1995 (consistent with encounter data). The first clinical date of June 30, 1994, was probably incorrectly entered and should be the date of the third shot: June 30, 1995. Inconsistent dates are a common problem in clinical data sets.

Decision rules about how to handle inconsistent data should be applied uniformly within a variable (e.g., birthdate); however they may be different across variables (e.g., birthdate and immunization date).

The purpose of checking on data quality is to identify potential data problems that could affect your results before beginning analysis. Problems that are identified during this process of "cleaning the data" must be resolved. Often this requires that a judgment be made by the analytical team about how to resolve the problem. All decisions should be documented for others to understand how the analysis was conducted. Documentation should be thorough enough that the analysis is "reproducible" (i.e., so that it could be carried out with exactly the same results by another analytic team). Because considerable resources can be expended in data cleaning, especially in consistency checks, it is advisable to consider the data elements that will be used in any analysis and focus on cleaning those variables for which accuracy is most important. Cleaning is an iterative process. As analysis proceeds, additional cleaning tasks will have to be undertaken. At this early step, you are trying to address the most obvious problems. In the following sections, we discuss some common approaches to resolving data-quality problems.

Missing Data Problems. Missing data problems occur for a variety of reasons and understanding the reason is important for determining whether bias (a systematic tendency to overestimate or underestimate the quantity of interest) is a potential problem. Possible reasons why data may be missing include

- The information was *not recorded*. For example, the child had an immunization, but this was not recorded in the medical record.

- A survey participant *refused* to answer the question. For instance, information on income is considered sensitive by many respondents and questions about household income are frequently skipped.

- An answer was *miscoded* by an interviewer or data entry clerk. This problem often shows up as an out-of-range value.

- Part of a medical record was *lost*. For example, a laboratory slip with test results is not found in the medical record and could not be recorded.

Table 6.10 illustrates the type of questions analysts should pose when evaluating the extent and nature of missing data problems.

Two main choices exist for dealing with subjects who having partially missing information:

- Exclude the observations and analyze only those cases with all needed information; or

- Use a variety of techniques to fill in the missing information.

One question you should ask about any analysis that already has been conducted as well as the data files you work with is, "How were missing data handled?" This is important because the approach that was taken to fix the missing data problem may significantly affect the results and thus the conclusions you might draw. One sign of a good analysis is proper documentation of how missing data were handled.

The fundamental analytic task is how to address the problem introduced by having missing data. This can be complex and consultation with a statistician is recommended. Four common approaches to this problem are

- **Exclude observations (e.g., individuals) without complete data:** This choice is frequently the default option on statistical software packages. This approach may be reasonable if very few data are missing and if the data appear to be missing at random (i.e., without any discernible pattern). If data are not missing at random, this approach is likely to introduce significant biases. For example, if we excluded from the analysis all children whose parents did not report their income, we might get a biased understanding of the relationship between income and the receipt of immunizations. To reduce the likelihood of bias, one of the following three

Table 6.10

Questions to Pose About Missing Data

What data are missing?

How often are data missing? Is more than 5 percent of data for key variables missing?

What are possible reasons that explain why they are missing? Are the data missing randomly or systematically (e.g., are there patterns of missing data, such as high-income people not responding)?

How critical are the missing data to the analyses?

Can I ignore the missing data problem or do I need to fix it?

If I do not fix the missing data problem, what are the implications for my results (e.g., bias)?

"replacement" approaches is generally recommended when there are large amounts of missing data or the data do not appear to be missing randomly.

- **Impute a value for missing data:** Using this method, the missing information is filled in using an analytic technique such as (1) substituting answers given by similar persons in the group for the missing information (i.e., hot deck imputation), (2) using the mean value of the missing variable for the sample (i.e., mean imputation), (3) using a predicted value based on a regression model that includes all available information (i.e., regression imputation), or (4) making an assumption that missing data are equivalent to a particular answer (i.e., cold deck imputation). A variable that suffers from significant missing data problems can also be dropped from an analysis if another variable is available that is an adequate substitute.

- **Weight the sample to account for nonresponse:** These methods are generally used when the entire observation is missing, such as is the case for surveys with nonrespondents. The approach assigns different *nonresponse weights* to each observation in a way that attempts to make the actual sample who responded to the survey closely reflect the total population from which the sample was drawn. This may mean "inflating" some observations (e.g., those for groups of individuals who were less likely to respond) and "deflating" other observations (e.g., those for groups who were more likely to respond). Such nonresponse weights are related to the sampling weights discussed above.

- **Use modeling techniques for partially missing data:** In this approach, a model or relationship between nonmissing and missing data is developed to explain the missing data and estimates are derived from the available data to use in place of missing data. These techniques are more flexible than the other approaches and you can test the effect of assumptions made on the results. However, these techniques generally require making more assumptions than the others.

The techniques used to address problems of missing data also apply to the issues of response and nonresponse bias, which will be discussed below. Because it is rarely the case that all of the information needed for an analysis is available, addressing the problem of missing data is a critical part of constructing the analysis data base. The technical summary description of any analysis should include an explicit discussion of the approach used to handle missing data and an explanation of resulting modifications to statistical techniques. In using survey data that were previously corrected and that contain sampling weights, you should understand the construction of the weights and the adequacy of adjustment for nonresponse. Typically, weights correct for certain types of nonresponse and may not specifically apply to your problem.[4] A sensitivity analysis that compares and contrasts the results based on applying different missing data techniques is an integral part of any complete analysis.

Errors in Measurement. The values for most variables contain some error. Some portion of the error is "noise," in that it represents random, not systematic, fluctuations in measurements. For example, if you weighed yourself four times during the day you might get four different values because your body weight fluctuates with food and fluid intake and the measurement instrument (your scale) may also produce somewhat different numbers. Other types of measurement error are "systematic," meaning that a value is routinely underestimated or overestimated (e.g., your scale at home always gives a weight 5 to 10 pounds lower than the scale in your doctor's office). Systematic errors pose a greater problem than random errors because of their potential to introduce bias into any analysis.

If errors occur randomly—there is no particular pattern to who gives an inaccurate answer or to the type of person whose laboratory test is misinterpreted—we can tolerate the error, knowing that it decreases our confidence in the results. On average, these errors tend to cancel each other out, since some will be too high and others too low. We are more concerned with measurement errors that occur nonrandomly, since the error is consistently in one direction and is persistent. For example, people with poor health habits (e.g., those who smoke, drink to excess, or fail to exercise) may be more likely to report inaccurate answers to questions about those behaviors than people with good health habits. If we do not account for likely problems in reporting, we could draw erroneous conclusions about the extent of health problems in the population.

Errors in measurement can occur in several ways. It is important to understand the likelihood that measurement errors exist in the data set, the probable source of those errors, and the problems you are likely to encounter in analyzing data that include errors. Measurement error can occur because

- A question was poorly worded;

- The respondent could not accurately remember the information requested;

- The respondent deliberately provided inaccurate information;

- The exact information was not available and so another variable was used instead (i.e., a proxy measure);

---

[4]Some data files contain sampling weights that adjust for nonresponse. You should review the file documentation to understand what types of missing data the weights correct for.

- A coding system may not include categories for all services provided or diagnoses observed, resulting in some codes being used inappropriately;

- A laboratory test was conducted or interpreted inaccurately; or

- A diagnostic test result was recorded inaccurately.

The solution to measurement error depends on the nature of the problem. Wherever possible, it is advisable to think about possible sources of bias during the design stage of data collection. At this point, you can take steps to reduce the likelihood of bias, for example, by how you sample from the population or by the way in which a survey is administered. However, in many cases, existing data are used to conduct an analysis (referred to as secondary data analysis). Because the data have already been collected, you will not be able to influence the potential for bias that may occur during the data collection stage. Consequently, you may need to consider ways to correct bias problems, if they exist, during the analysis stage.

Analyses of cost data are likely to use econometric models that rely on the assumption that the variables are free from errors. There are no formal tests for determining whether errors exist in cost data sets; however, econometricians use a variety of solutions to correct for likely errors. These include

- Inverse least squares;

- The two-group method;

- The three-group method;

- Weighted regression;

- Durbin's ranking method;

- Instrumental variables; and

- Maximum likelihood.

For more information about these methods to address bias, see Pindyck and Rubinfield (1991) or Koutsoyiannis (1985). Consulting a statistician is recommended as well.

The next section addresses the various sources of measurement error that result in bias.

Common Sources of Bias. Bias occurs when the individuals on whom data are collected, the groups that are being compared, or particular variables differ in a systematic way from the population from which they were sampled. Bias can be introduced at any step in the collection, coding, and analysis of data. Several common sources of bias are described below:

Selection bias refers to how people select into the group that you are analyzing. For example, in making comparisons among groups (e.g., enrollees in a FFS health plan compared to those in an HMO health plan), you often encounter the problem that the groups are not comparable because different types of people have chosen to be members of each group. Because HMOs tend to have tighter controls on utilization of care, sicker patients might be more likely to select into a FFS plan. If enrollees in the HMO plan have lower utilization rates, this may be because they are healthier than those in the FFS plan. We care about selection bias principally because it affects our ability to draw accurate conclusions, such as whether plan type affects utilization.

Say you are interested in evaluating whether a new treatment program for substance abuse is effective and you decide to let people volunteer for either the treatment program or the control group. This type of study design is "observational" or "nonexperimental," since you, the investigator, do not have control over the assignment of people to the comparison groups (treatment or control). When you do have control over assignment, the design is experimental. A common way to assign individuals is by randomization and the good statistical properties of the resulting design explain the popularity of randomized controlled trials.

In an observational study, if you find that the treatment group had better outcomes than the control group, you do not know whether people who decided to enter treatment were more highly motivated to improve than the volunteer control group or whether the treatment program was really effective. More subtle forms of selection bias occur regularly in the health care system—who self-selects treatment from specialists rather than generalists, who chooses to wear or not to wear seat belts, who seeks health services for acute, self-limiting conditions—and each selection choice affects what we can conclude using nonexperimental or observational data. Selection bias is a concern any time a group has been formed other than through random assignment or a random sorting process.

Response bias occurs primarily in surveys when individuals systematically inflate or deflate their answers. It can occur either intentionally (e.g., reporting fewer cigarettes smoked than actual, reporting more exercise than actual, or underreporting earned income) or unintentionally (e.g., inaccurate recall of when an individual last visited a physician).

Nonresponse bias occurs primarily in surveys when individuals choose not to participate. If nonresponse occurs randomly, that is, if the characteristics of individuals who do and who do not respond to a survey are similar, nonresponse is less problematic. If the failure to respond is not random (e.g., wealthy individuals choose not to participate), bias is introduced into the data set.

Omitted variable bias occurs when an important variable is left out of the analysis, either because the analyst did not include it or because data were not available on that variable. For example, if you were trying to predict the relationship between individual characteristics and low-birthweight births, and you failed to include whether or not the mother was a smoker in the analysis, other factors (e.g., income) might appear more important than they actually are. This is because they are capturing some of the effect on the response (low birthweight) that would otherwise be attributed to the omitted variable (smoking status).

Attrition bias occurs when particular subsets of individuals leave a group at different rates from other individuals (e.g., sicker people leave as a result of death or sicker people leave to go to other health plans that provide greater access). If you are comparing the same groups in multiple time periods, the characteristics of individuals in the groups may change because some people may be more likely to drop out than others (e.g., those who are very sick) and the change in the mix of group characteristics may influence the results more than the intervention you are trying to evaluate. This problem can occur under any study design.

Attrition often occurs when comparing two alternative treatments for a condition. Say, for example, that old people are more likely to have worse health outcomes than young people. You are comparing treatment A with treatment B and randomly assign people to either treatment group. As it turns out, neither treatment works (i.e., neither treatment produces better health outcomes). But, if more old people drop out of Group A than out of Group B, it might appear that the treatment provided to Group A is better. In fact, because Group B has a higher proportion of old people, the average health outcome score for the entire group is worse as compared with Group A, which has a lower proportion of old people.

The Hawthorne effect refers to differences in behavior or answers to questions that are a direct result of the fact that someone is being studied or observed. People may behave more responsibly than they would otherwise (e.g., obtaining routine screening tests or preventive services on schedule) or may give answers they think the researcher wants (i.e., socially desirable responses).

Approaches to Dealing with Bias. The way in which a study is conducted (i.e., design phase decisions) can reduce the potential for bias in the data. For example, randomized controlled trials reduce opportunities for bias because individuals participating in such studies are randomly assigned to the intervention that is under investigation. Random assignment (if it is maintained throughout the life of the study) eliminates problems such as selection bias.

Similarly, techniques designed to ensure high rates of response to surveys (e.g., telephone follow-up to mail surveys) can significantly reduce nonresponse bias.

However, for many analysts, the data will have already been collected and opportunities to reduce bias during data collection will not be possible. Thus, the discussion that follows focuses primarily on techniques to deal with bias during the analysis stage. Table 6.11 summarizes the main points of the discussion.

Selection bias can be dealt with in a variety of ways. All the techniques attempt to identify the source or the nature of the bias and then use analytic methods to "correct" for the problem. Selection bias is common and important in setting reimbursement rates for traditional indemnity insurance plans and capitated health plans. Several studies have shown that "favorable" selection exists in managed care plans—that is, such plans tend to attract healthier enrollees (Billi et al., 1993; Diehr et al., 1993; Davidson et al., 1992; van Vliet and van de Ven, 1992; Riley et al., 1991; and Miller and Luft, 1994). In response, techniques have been suggested to *risk-adjust* employer contributions to insurance plans to reflect differences in health risks and costs (Robinson et al., 1991; Bowen

Table 6.11

Approaches to Dealing with Bias

Source of Bias	Potential Solutions	
	Design Phase	Analysis Phase
Selection	Sampling method (random sampling)	Risk adjustment
Response	Design of survey questionnaire Interview technique (e.g., face-to-face) Length of questionnaire Sponsorship by credible organization	Inflate/deflate responses Define different cutpoints
Nonresponse	Interview method (e.g., telephone or mail) Sponsorship by credible organization Length of questionnaire Repeated follow-up	Exclude observations with missing data, if similar to complete cases Impute missing value (e.g., assign mean value) Weight sample to account for non-response Model relationship between missing and nonmissing data
Omitted variable	Careful specification of data elements and analytic model	Add missing variable, if available Use proxy or instrumental variable
Attrition	Structured follow-up Financial incentives to participate Continue to collect data on those who exit the study	Intention to treat analysis Impute missing data
Hawthorne effect	Use placebo Blind researcher and patient to receipt of intervention	Inflate/deflate responses Define different cutpoints

and Slavin, 1991). Conceptually, the idea is to predict prospectively the expenditures of a group of individuals enrolling in a health plan using characteristics that are known at the time of enrollment (e.g., age, gender, health status, and prior utilization). There is general agreement that the ability to predict such behavior a priori is limited (Newhouse et al., 1989); therefore, techniques that employ post-hoc adjustments may also be required. Please refer to Chapter Nine for a detailed discussion of risk adjustment.

Response bias presents a particularly difficult problem for analysis because information has been systematically altered, generally by those individuals about whom we are most interested (e.g., smokers or heavy drinkers). There are no easy answers to dealing with response bias, but a couple of approaches could be used during data analysis. First, if you have information about "real" patterns (e.g., from some other study that collected data using techniques other than respondent self-report), you could inflate or deflate answers accordingly. This requires that you believe that the pattern of under- or overreporting is consistent. Second, being aware of tendencies to change answers, you might set cutpoints (i.e., thresholds for identifying heavy and light drinkers) differently to take these reporting problems into account.

Nonresponse bias can be addressed using the techniques discussed above in the section on handling missing data.

Omitted variable bias can be solved only by adding the missing variable into the analysis. In some cases, the variable that you need is not available and you may have to construct one that serves as a proxy for the missing information. The problem of omitted variable bias can be quite subtle because you may be unaware that an important independent variable is missing.

Attrition bias must be dealt with first by determining the extent and nature of attrition. If you are comparing two groups, you can begin by examining whether those who did not complete the observation period are different from those who did complete it, particularly on characteristics that might affect the outcome of interest.

For example, if you were comparing the outcomes of two different drug abuse treatment programs, you would look at whether those who dropped out of treatment in the two programs were different from those who stayed in terms of the severity of their drug use, the length of time they had been abusing drugs, the presence of any comorbid conditions (e.g., mental disorder), age, gender, and so on. If dropout rates are low (e.g., less than 10 percent) or if those who drop out are no different from those who stay in, you may be less concerned about attrition bias. However, if dropouts result in the groups becoming more different at the end of the observation period than they were in the beginning, you need to worry about bias related to attrition.

The most conservative method for dealing with attrition bias is by doing an "intention to treat" analysis, that is, to include in the analysis everyone who began the intervention (e.g., treatment protocol) and compare outcomes for the two groups regardless of whether people stayed in the treatment. This approach is possible if you have been able to continue collecting data on people who drop out of treatment. If you have evidence that attrition bias is a problem and you cannot do an intention to treat analysis, then you should find another way to control for the bias. Some of the techniques listed under missing data will apply (discussed above), such as imputing outcomes for missing observations based on outcomes for similar persons who remained in the analysis.

The Hawthorne effect is a difficult problem to address because the fact of being observed or measured can change people's behavior. One way to deal with this is to select the least-intrusive data source; surveys or direct observation tend to be more intrusive than abstracting information from existing records. Another approach is to use a placebo (either treatment or survey instrument) that blinds the participants to who is receiving treatment and who is being studied. One can also treat this as a special case of a response bias and apply the same analytic techniques for dealing with the problem.

Before beginning your analysis, you should have your proposed study reviewed by experts in the area that you are studying. This process can serve to identify possible sources of bias. If your study involves collecting data, design solutions may be suggested to avoid bias. If you believe bias exists and no solution is available to correct for the bias, at a minimum you should try to identify the direction and the magnitude of the bias to say how your results might be affected by the bias (i.e., an estimate is too low or too high). For example, if you believe that heavy drinkers are likely to underreport their consumption of alcohol, you would report that your estimates were likely to be lower than the true rate of alcohol consumption in the population.

Once you have formulated the study question, selected the data sources, and constructed the analytic data set with as few problems or errors as possible, you are ready to do some preliminary analyses. It should be clear that the preparatory steps are both time-consuming and critical. Rarely should you proceed directly to analyzing data without having gone through these preparatory steps. The time taken in preparing to do an analysis will save considerable trouble later. In planning to do analyses, it is important to allow sufficient time to undertake these preliminary steps.

A SAMPLER OF ANALYTIC TECHNIQUES

It is beyond the scope of this book to describe all of the possible analytic techniques that could be used to explore answers to questions based on the range of data available. We will endeavor, therefore, simply to highlight some of the most common analytic techniques, indicating the types of questions and data to which they are most often applied. Analysis can be divided into three major categories:

- Description;

- Inference; and

- Prediction.

We will discuss specific techniques within these major groups.

Description

Descriptive analysis involves examining data in tabular, graphical, or numerical form to determine whether there are any important patterns in the data set, such as relationships between variables.

- Univariate analysis refers to statistics performed on a single variable (e.g., counts, frequency distributions, and histograms).

- Bivariate analysis concerns pairs of variables (e.g., cross-tabulation, correlation, and scatter plots).

Descriptive analysis is done to provide a context within which other information can be considered and is the first step in any analysis. Often, descriptive analysis is used to identify potential data problems that were not detected in cleaning the data. It facilitates comparisons between the current analysis and other related work that has been done.[5] However, descriptive analysis does not allow inference from the sample back to the population, as it does not involve the type of probabilistic reasoning required to draw conclusions. Simple descriptive statistics also do not control for the effect of other factors that may explain the observed outcome.

Usually the first step is to determine the types of variables to be used in the analysis. This determination is important, since the technique chosen for analysis depends on the type of variables involved. Variables may be divided into two basic types:

- **Quantitative:** the values of a quantitative variable lie on a numerical scale (e.g., temperature); and

---

[5]You should compare the descriptive statistics from your study to previous studies of the same problem, if they exist.

- **Qualitative:** the values of a qualitative variable do not lie on a numerical scale (e.g., insured or uninsured and male or female).

Quantitative variables may be divided further into those that are

- **Discrete:** variables where large gaps exist between the possible values. An example of discrete quantitative variable is years of school completed; and

- **Continuous:** variables where no gaps exist between possible values. An example of a continuous quantitative variable is blood pressure.

Sometimes the division between discrete and continuous variables is unclear, because, for example, a patient may complete only a half year of school. In the blood pressure example, technically gaps may exist between blood pressure readings, as the blood pressure machine can measure the pressure only to a certain degree of accuracy, say the third decimal place. However, to determine variable type, you should consider theoretically whether the possible values of the variable correspond to a range of values on a number line, or to distinct values on the number line. The former type of variable is continuous and the latter is discrete. Often a discrete variable that has many possible values is treated as a continuous variable in analysis (e.g., age).

Qualitative variables, which are also known as categorical variables, may be further divided into those that are

- **Ordinal:** variables where a natural ordering to the values or categories exists. An example of an ordinal qualitative variable is a patient satisfaction scale consisting of the values "extremely dissatisfied," "dissatisfied," "neutral," "satisfied," and "extremely satisfied;" and

- **Nominal:** variables where a natural ordering to the values does not exist. An example of a nominal qualitative variable is insurance status with values such as "uninsured," "self-insured," and "privately insured."

A particularly important type of nominal qualitative variable is a binary one, that is, one with two outcomes. For example, the answer to "Do you have insurance?" has two possible outcomes: yes or no. This variable is binary or dichotomous and is often recoded to a 1 for yes and a 0 for no, or vice versa. The analyst must distinguish between the meaning of the values of a variable and numeric codes that these values have been assigned for ease in data entry or computer work.

The second step is to describe the values assigned to each variable in the analysis and how common each value is (referred to as the distribution of the values for key variables). The distribution of a single variable can be shown through frequencies and histograms. The distribution of a single variable as influenced by other variables can be shown through cross-tabs.

A *frequency* is a count of how many individuals have a particular value (male or female) of the variable of interest (gender). Frequency tables are appropriate for qualitative variables. They are also appropriate for quantitative variables that can take on a limited number of values or can be divided into discrete categories. Artificially dividing the variable into meaningful categories can also produce a useful frequency table. For example, the continuous variable age can be divided into the following categories:

- < age 18;
- age 18–35;
- age 36–50; and
- > age 50.

Table 6.12 contains an example of a frequency table for gender, which is a dichotomous, qualitative variable.

A *histogram* is simply a graphical representation of a frequency table. It is often easier to identify patterns in variables from pictures than from numeric summaries. Figure 6.1 below illustrates a histogram that summarizes the age variable.

Histograms for qualitative variables are also called bar charts. Often, histograms for quantitative or ordinal variables, that is, for variables whose categories have a natural ordering, are often compared with a symmetric bell-shaped (Normal, Gaussian) distribution. The histogram shown in Figure 6.1 does not have a bell-shaped distribution. This distribution is "skewed," which means that it has an asymmetric distribution with decreasing numbers of values trailing off to the right in the older age categories. If a variable is normally

Table 6.12

Sample Frequency Table for Gender

Values	Frequency	Cumulative Frequency	Percent	Cumulative Percent
Gender				
. (missing)	500	500	1.0	1.0
1 (male)	24,300	24,800	49.6	50.6
2 (female)	25,000	49,800	50.0	99.6
9 (unknown)	200	50,000	0.4	100.0

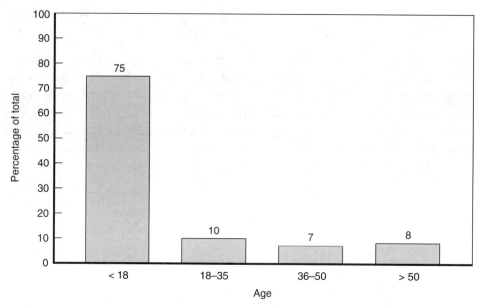

Figure 6.1—Sample Histogram for Age

distributed, certain types of analysis are facilitated. Often, an assumption of normality is required for a specific statistical technique to be applicable, so checking for normality is a good idea.[6]

A *cross-tab* (cross-tabulation) illustrates the relationship between two variables by showing the frequency with which combinations of values occur. This may be helpful for understanding whether certain groups as defined by one variable are more or less likely to have a particular characteristic (the second variable). In Table 6.13, for example, we see a bivariate descriptive analysis of income by insurance status for a random sample of U.S. residents. Persons in the high-income group are more likely to have private insurance, whereas persons in the low-income group are more likely to have Medicaid. Generally, cross-tabs are done showing column and row percentages so that you can understand the relative frequency for each element in the table. The table shows, for example, that 90 percent of those with high incomes have private insurance compared to 75 percent of those with medium incomes and 25 percent of those with low incomes. This table suggests that increasing income may be positively associated with having private insurance coverage. However, because cross-tabs do not control for other factors that may influence the observed relationship, they

---

[6]If normality does not exist, you should consult a statistician for advice on how to transform variables so that their distributions more closely approximate the normal curve.

Table 6.13

Sample Cross Tabulation for Income by Insurance Status

Income Group	Insurance Status			
	Private	Medicaid	Uninsured	Totals
High	9,000	0	1,000	10,000
Row %	(90)	(0)	(10)	(100)
Column %	(26)	(0)	(17)	(20)
Medium	22,500	3,000	4,500	30,000
Row %	(75)	(10)	(15)	(100)
Column %	(66)	(30)	(75)	(60)
Low	2,500	7,000	500	10,000
Row %	(25)	(70)	(5)	(100)
Column %	(7)	(70)	(8)	(20)
Totals	34,000	10,000	6,000	50,000
Row %	(68)	(20)	(12)	(100)
Column %	(100)	(100)	(100)	(100)

cannot be used to draw conclusions or inferences. These techniques are discussed in the next section.

Although examining key variables in graphical or tabular form is an important part of the initial analysis, the graphs or tables are often too numerous or complicated to describe and present. For quantitative variables, the next common step in a descriptive analysis is to summarize two aspects of the distribution of each variable: the center and the spread. There are several ways to measure both the center and spread of a variable. For a sample (i.e., a subset of the population), these numerical summaries of center and spread are known as statistics. Definitions of common summary statistics for a single variable are shown in Table 6.14.

Most of the measures shown in Table 6.14 are applicable only for quantitative variables. For a qualitative variable (except binary), the mode is usually reported as a measure of center and a condensed frequency table is presented to show the spread of the variable.

Most statistical packages have standard procedures for producing descriptive summaries of variables and often will produce more than one measure for both center and spread. Comparing different measures of the same dimension is often a useful exercise. For example, if the mean is very different from the median, the variable is usually skewed; that is, it has an asymmetric distribution that may produce analytic challenges. An example of this is income. The mean income in the United States in 1992 was $39,020 and the median income was $30,786 (Bureau of the Census, 1994). The mean value is higher than the median, since it is being influenced by households with extremely large incomes. Examining the graphical, tabular, and numerical patterns exhibited

Table 6.14

Definitions of Descriptive Statistics

Term	Definition
Measures of center	
Mean	The arithmetic average (sum of all the values divided by the number of units on which the value was observed). This is the most common way of summarizing the central value of a quantitative characteristic. However, this measure is sensitive to outliers (extreme values).
Mode	The most frequently observed value.
Median	The midpoint of the data (50 percent of values are higher than the median and 50 percent are lower than the median). This is also known as the 50th percentile. This measure is not sensitive to outliers.
Measures of spread	
Standard deviation	The square root of the average squared distance between each value and the mean. This is the most common way to summarize the spread of a variable. However, this measure is sensitive to outliers.
Range	The difference between the maximum and the minimum values. This measure is sensitive to outliers.
Interquartile range	The difference between the 75th (i.e., 75 percent of values are below this point) and 25th percentiles. This measure is not sensitive to outliers.

by a variable alone and in relation to other variables will help you understand your key variables and simple relationships among those variables so that you may select the appropriate analytic technique for answering your question.

Inference

As discussed above, descriptive statistics are used to summarize variables, either graphically or numerically, and either singly or jointly. Descriptive summaries are an informative first task in a statistical analysis. The second two tasks in a statistical analysis are inference and prediction.

- Inference determines what we might conclude from the sample that we have available to analyze about the population that we wish to learn more about (that is, the population we would like to generalize our sample results to).

- Prediction considers "what we might expect." When we ask, "What we do expect?" we mean in the future, what values might certain variables take on.

Both inference and prediction contain some level of uncertainty, since we are basing our conclusions on information drawn from a sample. We are able to measure this uncertainty when we know the chance or probability that any member of the population has of being in our sample. That is, we can make inferences based only on probability samples. Probability provides the bridge between the sample and the population. Thus, although our sample is not a complete picture of the population, we can determine the extent to which the sample is likely to differ from the underlying population and, therefore, the degree to which we believe the sample is representative of the entire population.

This section discusses the two major strategies in inference:

• Estimation; and

• Statistical hypothesis testing.

These two approaches are discussed in the context of a single quantitative variable that can take on a range of values, such as health care expenditures or blood pressure (continuous or variable). The approaches extend to univariate analysis of different types of variables, such as discrete counts, and to the combination of variables, such as the examination of two categorical variables. A good reference for these extensions is Snedecor and Cochran (1980).

Estimation. Suppose that we want to know the average annual expenditure for medical services of people enrolled in a health plan. It would be expensive to gather this information on everyone and then calculate the average annual expenditure for the entire population of enrollees. Thus, we will estimate the average annual expenditure using a sample of enrolled persons, and, furthermore, we will gauge how good our estimate is in relation to the true population value. Estimation is the first task of inference.

We begin by drawing a simple random sample of 1,000 people from the population of enrollees. Recall that by a *simple random sample*, we mean that every member of the population has an equal chance of being sampled. As discussed in the previous section on descriptive analysis, we summarize the sample's expenditures by calculating the sample mean (average) expenditure and the sample standard deviation. Suppose the sample mean is $797 and the sample standard deviation is $3,896.[7]

What we would like to know is how close this estimate, the sample mean annual expenditure, is to the true population mean annual expenditure (i.e., the average annual expenditure of *all* enrolled people). The sample mean annual expenditure for any sample depends upon the group of people who were sampled; a different value might have been obtained on a different sample of people. We reflect the randomness of our sampling procedure by providing an interval estimate rather than the single sample average of $797 (a point estimate).

---

[7]These are the observed values for the individual deductible subgroup in the RAND Health Insurance Experiment (HIE) (Newhouse and the Insurance Experiment Group, 1993). In fact, analyses of expenditures are usually performed on a log scale to correct for skewed distributions, but we use dollars here to simplify the example.

With a random sample size of 1,000 and a sample mean of $797 and a standard deviation of $3,896, the range of values would be between $556 and $1,038. We call this range of possible mean annual expenditure values a *confidence interval*.

Attached to our confidence interval is the *confidence level,* or the degree to which we believe the interval contains the true population mean. The $556 to $1,038 range has a confidence level of 95 percent. The complete confidence interval statement for this interval is, "We are 95 percent confident that the average annual expenditure of the population lies between $556 and $1,038." By 95 percent confident we mean that, if we repeated our sampling procedure over and over again (a hypothetical exercise, since we only draw one sample in reality), on average, 95 percent of the confidence intervals we would construct would contain the true average annual expenditure of the population.

This interval estimate is constructed using

1. The *standard deviation*, which tells us how much annual expenditure varies across enrollees;

2. The *sample size*, which tells us how much information we have on which to base our estimate; and

3. The *confidence level*, which tells us how strongly we can believe our interval.

The narrower the confidence interval, the more information it gives us. For example, compare a confidence interval of $100 to $2,000 with the confidence interval of $556 to $1,038. The latter interval is more precise as it indicates a smaller range of values in which we believe the mean annual expenditure for the population lies.

How might we narrow a confidence interval? Consider the three components that are used to construct confidence intervals. We cannot change the first component, the standard deviation, as this value depends on the variation in annual expenditures among enrollees, which is not within our control.[8] We can change the second component, the sample size. Increasing the sample size will narrow the confidence interval. Intuitively, the more information we have, that is, the larger sample we have, the more precisely we can estimate the population mean annual expenditure and the narrower our confidence interval will be.

---

[8]The standard deviation could be made narrower by selecting a more homogeneous population, such as only children or only persons ages 18–44. However, since we are interested in the average annual expenditure of all enrollees, we cannot restrict analysis to such a subgroup without possibly incurring bias.

Our estimate of the population mean annual expenditure is the sample mean annual expenditure and the error in this estimate decreases with the square root of the sample size. In fact, the standard deviation of the sample mean annual expenditures is equal to the standard deviation of the individual annual expenditures divided by the square root of the sample size. This quantity is known as the *standard error.* In our example, the standard error is $123 ($3,936 divided by the square root of 1,000). A 95 percent confidence interval is approximately the sample mean plus and minus twice the standard error (see the following equation). In our example, $797 plus or minus $246 is approximately equal to $556 to $1,038.

Confidence interval (C. I.) formulas

$$\text{Standard error (s.e.)} = \frac{\text{standard deviation}}{\sqrt{\text{sample size}}}$$

95 percent C. I. lower bound = mean − 1.96*s.e.

95 percent C. I. upper bound = mean + 1.96*s.e.

For a 90 percent C. I., replace 1.96 by 1.65

For an 80 percent C. I., replace 1.96 by 1.28

We can also change the third component, the confidence level. If we are content to decrease the strength of our belief in our confidence interval, say from 95 percent to 90 percent, we can narrow the confidence interval. The usual convention is to set the confidence level at 95 percent. Table 6.15 shows the tradeoff between the components in a confidence interval, assuming that the sample mean annual expenditure is $797 and the standard deviation is constant at $3,936.

The table shows that to cut in half the width of the confidence interval, we must quadruple the sample size. For example, to go from a confidence interval that is

Table 6.15

**Tradeoff Between Components in a
Confidence Interval**

Sample Size	Confidence Level	Confidence Interval
1,000	95%	$556 to $1,038
1,500	95%	$600 to $994
2,000	95%	$626 to $968
4,000	95%	$676 to $917
1,000	90%	$594 to $1,000
1,500	90%	$632 to $962
2,000	80%	$685 to $909

$482 wide ($556 to $1,038) to one that is $241 wide ($676 to $917) at a confidence level of 95 percent, we must increase our sample size from 1,000 to 4,000.

One task in designing a study is to determine the sample size. If estimation is a study goal, a *precision analysis* will help determine the sample size. A precision analysis calculates the sample size required to construct a confidence interval of a certain width. Such a calculation requires choosing a confidence level and assuming that the standard deviation is a particular value. We often do not know the standard deviation but we may have a range of possible values from previous studies. For example, suppose we want to construct a 95 percent confidence interval that is $482 wide. If we assume that the standard deviation is $3,936, we would need a sample of size 1,000 as shown in Table 6.15. Alternatively, if we assume that the standard deviation is $4,500, our sample size would have to be 1,340 to maintain the same width. Enlarging the sample allows us to overcome the increased variability in enrollee annual expenditure. However, increasing the sample size will increase the cost of the study, which may affect other components of the study, such as additional data collection per person.

Hypothesis Testing. The other major strategy in inference is statistical hypothesis testing, which answers a specific question rather than providing an estimate of a particular quantity. Consider a sample of patients who have high blood pressure. We measure each patient's blood pressure before administering a new drug and after. As discussed in the previous design section, each patient is acting as his or her own control in this pre-post design. We quantify the effect of the treatment as the difference between the pre-treatment and post-treatment blood pressure measurements.

$$\text{Treatment effect} = \text{pre-treatment blood pressure measure} \\ - \text{post-treatment blood pressure measure}$$

If we were to choose the optimal design for a study of a new drug, we might well use a randomized controlled trial. However, the pre-post design is chosen to make the discussion of hypothesis testing easier to explain because we have a single group of patients and a single statistic for each patient (the treatment effect).

We conclude that the treatment works if we observe a large decrease in blood pressure for a large number of patients in our sample after they have received the new drug (that is, a large positive effect). The theory of hypothesis testing helps us determine how large a decrease, and in how many patients we must observe a decrease, before we draw such a conclusion. The theory also helps us gauge the strength of our conclusion.

Suppose we observe, on average across our sample of patients, a decrease in blood pressure after the treatment. Even though we observe this decrease, we must question whether the decrease is attributable to the treatment or just to chance. Perhaps the decrease we have observed is because of the random nature of our sampling procedure. It might be that even though the treatment does not have an effect on blood pressure, some people have a decrease in blood pressure over time and others have an increase. By chance, we may have selected a sample of primarily the former type of people. With a statistical hypothesis test, we hope to distinguish between an average decrease in blood pressure resulting from sampling variability and an average decrease resulting from a treatment effect (i.e., the drug actually works).

To conduct a formal statistical test of this question, we construct a null hypothesis (often represented symbolically as H_0), which is usually that no difference exists. In our example, the null hypothesis would be that the treatment does not reduce blood pressure. We also construct an alternative, or study, hypothesis (often represented as H_1). In our example, the alternative hypothesis would be that the treatment does decrease blood pressure. Hypotheses are constructed based on theory and past research.

H_0 = treatment does not reduce blood pressure (i.e., there is no treatment effect).
H_1 = treatment does reduce blood pressure (i.e., there is a treatment effect).

The statistical test involves assessing whether what we observed is consistent with the null hypothesis of no treatment effect. If it is not, we reject the null hypothesis because the data are strong enough to cast considerable doubt on the null hypothesis being true. That is, the data suggest that the observed treatment effect is real and not simply due to chance. We conclude that the observed reduction in blood pressure resulting from the treatment is "statistically significant." Our conclusion based on this empirical evidence is that the treatment is effective and decreases blood pressure.

If the data are consistent with the null hypothesis—that the treatment had no effect—we do not reject the null hypothesis and conclude that we do not have enough evidence to cast doubt upon the null. We do not necessarily accept the null hypothesis that the treatment is ineffective, only that we do not have sufficient empirical evidence to conclude that the treatment is effective. Thus, the two possible conclusions of a statistical hypothesis test are that we reject the null hypothesis or that we do not reject the null hypothesis.

In doing a statistical test of the hypothesis, we base our conclusion on a sample of the data rather than on the entire population. Consequently, we may make

Table 6.16

Possible Results of a Hypothesis Test

	Decision	
State of the World	Do not reject H_0 (conclude that evidence is insufficient to deem treatment effective)	Reject H_0 (conclude that treatment is effective)
H_0 is true (treatment does not reduce blood pressure, i.e., is ineffective)	Correct decision Probability = $1 - \alpha$	Type I error Probability = α = significance level of the test
H_0 is false (treatment does reduce blood pressure, i.e., is effective)	Type II error Probability = β	Correct decision Probability = $1 - \beta$ = power of the test

one of two types of errors (see Table 6.16). The first error, known as *Type I error*, is made if we conclude that the treatment is effective in reducing blood pressure (reject H_0) when it really is ineffective (H_0 is true). We fix the probability of this error (α), also called the significance level of the test, before conducting the test. A common value for the significance level is 5 percent. The second error we may commit, known as a *Type II error*, occurs if we conclude that insufficient evidence exists to conclude that the treatment is effective (do not reject H_0) when it actually does (H_0 is false). The size of the probability of a Type II error (β) depends on the specific effect that the treatment has. Hypothesis tests are generally constructed so that the Type II error is minimized.

Suppose that we observe a large average decrease in blood pressure in our sample. Our conclusion is that "we reject the null hypothesis of no treatment effect at a significance level of 5 percent." Had we observed a smaller average decrease, we might still have rejected the null. Can we be more precise in the way we present the strength of our evidence against the null hypothesis?

The *p-value* for a test is the probability that we might observe a decrease in blood pressure larger than the decrease we did observe if the treatment had no effect, that is, if the null hypothesis was true.

The p-value is a measure of the strength of the evidence against the null hypothesis H_0. The smaller the p-value, the stronger the evidence against the null hypothesis, since the decrease we observed in our data or an even larger decrease would be extremely unlikely to have resulted by chance (that is, if the null hypothesis were true). P-values less than 5 percent, the common significance level of the test, indicate that we should reject the null. Because p-values are a continuous measure, they give us more information than the decision to reject or not reject the null hypothesis.

A common error is to interpret the p-value as the probability that the null is true. This interpretation is incorrect as the null hypothesis is either true or not true, and the p-value simply tells us the strength of our evidence against it.

Another piece of evidence that we can gather from our data is a confidence interval for the average decrease in blood pressure which, unlike the p-value, is in the units of the outcome variable (e.g., blood pressure or mm Hg). As a result, confidence intervals are thought by some to be more informative than a hypothesis test. In presenting results, it is best to include both the hypothesis test and associated confidence interval, as well as the descriptive statistics for the variable being examined, such as the sample mean and standard error. We now demonstrate conducting a statistical hypothesis test using another example.

Presume that our study objective is to test whether a difference exists between Canada and the United States in the percentage of patients who receive coronary angiography.

H_0 = no difference exists between the two counties in the rates of coronary angiography.

H_1 = a difference exists between the two counties in the rates of coronary angiography.

In the example shown in Table 6.17, 5 percent of Canadian patients compared to 11 percent of U.S. patients undergoing coronary angiography were age 75 or older. The p-value for the difference is less than 0.001 (0.1 percent), meaning that the null hypothesis of no difference in the proportion of elderly undergoing this procedure in the United States and Canada can be rejected strongly, since 0.1 percent is much less than the standard significance level of 5 percent. The 95 percent confidence interval is shown in parentheses—3 to 7 percent around

Table 6.17

Proportion of Patients Undergoing Coronary Angiography in Canada and the United States by Selected Demographic Characteristics

	Canada	United States
Age	(Confidence interval)	
≤ 59	49 (45–53)	42 (39–45)
60–74	46 (42–50)	47 (44–50)
≥ 75	5 (3–7)**	11 (10–13)
Female	28 (24–32)*	35 (31–40)

SOURCE: McGlynn et al. (1994).

$**p < 0.001; *p = 0.023.$

the observed number of 5 percent for Canada and 10 to 13 percent around the 11 percent observed in the United States. The fact that the two confidence intervals do not overlap, that is, they do not share any common values, is also an indication that the Canadian percentage is significantly different from the American percentage.

The proportion of women undergoing the procedure in the United States and Canada is also shown. Although we can reject the null hypothesis that there is no difference between the two countries in the proportion of women who receive the procedure, the evidence is less strong than that for the age test ($p = 0.023$ for gender compared to $p = 0.001$ for age); however, it is still well below the traditional value of $p = 0.05$.

The *power of a test* is the probability that we correctly conclude that the treatment has an effect on blood pressure when the treatment does actually have an effect. That is, power is the probability that we reject the null hypothesis when we should, i.e., when the alternative hypothesis is true. It is one minus the probability of a Type II error $(1 - \beta)$ as shown in Table 6.16.

The power depends on the specific size of the treatment effect—how much of a reduction in blood pressure occurs with treatment (i.e., which specific alternative hypothesis is true). Sample size can also affect the power: The larger the sample, the easier it is to distinguish between the null hypothesis and the true alternative hypothesis. A *power analysis* determines the size of the sample needed to attain a certain amount of power, usually 80 percent, with which to detect the difference between the null hypothesis and a specific alternative hypothesis. These calculations are conducted as a means to identify how large a sample must be selected to observe an effect. A power analysis may also be used with an existing data set to determine the power of the data to detect a significant difference.

Power calculations are usually carried out for a range of possible situations (e.g., different treatment effect sizes) so that the analyst can understand the sensitivity of the power for different alternative hypotheses. A power analysis for a hypothesis test is the analog of a precision analysis for a confidence interval, which was discussed above.

We return to our annual expenditure example drawn from the RAND HIE. Suppose that the average annual expenditure of all people enrolled in a particular health plan is $982 (this value was the level observed for the "free" insurance subgroup who faced no out-of-pocket expenditures in the RAND HIE). Because the number of observations for the health plan is large, the average annual expenditure is effectively known with certainty. We are interested in comparing the average annual expenditure of enrollees in a second health plan. We plan to draw a random sample of enrollees from the second health plan and use a statistical hypothesis test to determine if the average annual expenditure for the second group is significantly different from $982 (average annual expenditure of $982 is our null hypothesis).

- We hypothesize that the second health plan serves a healthier population whose average annual expenditure is $797 (average annual expenditure is $797 is our alternative hypothesis; this value was the level observed for the individual deductible subgroup in the RAND HIE).

- We also hypothesize that the standard deviation of annual expenditures in the second health plan is between $2,000 and $4,000, which is the range of standard deviations observed in the free insurance and individual deductible subgroups.

What size sample do we need to distinguish a difference in the average annual expenditure of the second health plan's enrollees from $982 with 80 percent power using a test with a 5 percent significance level? Since the hypotheses are informed guesses, it often makes sense to evaluate how the sample size requirements will vary under different assumptions, as shown in Table 6.18.

This analysis shows us that we need a random sample of at least 1,227 enrollees to distinguish an average annual expenditure of $797 from the known average of $982 in the first health plan with 80 percent power. We will have an 80 percent probability of rejecting the null hypothesis that the two average annual expenditures are equal if we conduct a 5 percent significance level test. We can see from this table that as the standard deviation increases (that is, as the variation in the annual expenditures of enrollees in the second health plan increases), we need a larger sample to achieve the same power. This occurs because additional enrollees in our sample are not as informative because of the additional variability among their annual expenditures.

Table 6.18

**Sample Size Required for 80 Percent Power
Based on Different Assumptions**

Average Annual Expenditure	Standard Deviation	Sample Size
$797	$2,000	1,227
$797	$3,000	2,761
$797	$4,000	4,908
$700	$2,000	528
$700	$3,000	1,188
$700	$4,000	2,112

If we hypothesize that the true average annual expenditure of enrollees in the second health plan is $700 rather than $797, we need a smaller sample size to distinguish this average from $982. The lower portion of the table shows that if the standard deviation is $2,000, we will need a random sample of only 528 enrollees as opposed to 1,227. As the alternative hypothesis moves farther away from the null hypothesis, we need a smaller sample size to distinguish among the two hypotheses with the same probability (power). We can see from Table 6.18 that the assumptions we make in our power analysis can have strong effects on the required sample size. The example underscores the need to conduct the calculations under a variety of assumptions and to draw a conservative conclusion.

Figure 6.2 shows the relationship between the significance level and power of a test and is the graphical representation of Table 6.16. The horizontal axis is the observed average annual expenditure of the random sample of enrollees in the second health plan. In this example, for ease of presentation, we will conduct a "one-sided" hypothesis test, in which we consider only if the second health plan's average is smaller than $982, the known average annual expenditure of the first health plan. The average at which we start to reject the null hypothesis (that the average annual expenditure in the second health plan is equal to $982) is known as the critical value of the test. This critical value is smaller than $982, since we must take into account the natural variability in annual expenditures and we do not want to make a Type I error too often (i.e., reject the null hypothesis when in fact the null is true, which in this example would mean that we

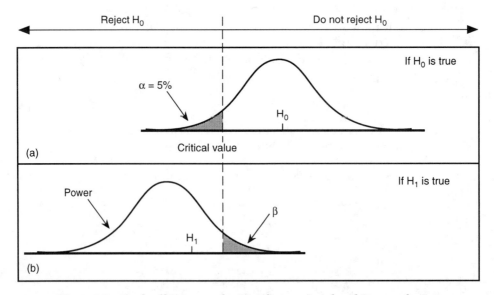

Figure 6.2—Tradeoff Between the Significance Level and Power of a Test

conclude that the average annual expenditure in the second health plan is smaller than that of the first health plan, when in fact the two are the same).

The upper portion of Figure 6.2 shows the significance level of our hypothesis test to the left of the critical value or the probability that we commit a Type I error (denoted as α, generally set at 5 percent). It is the probability that we observe a sample average expenditure smaller than the critical value when the null hypothesis is true.

The lower portion shows the power of our test to the left of the critical value. It is the probability that we reject the null hypothesis when the alternative is true (denoted as $1 - \beta$ and equal to the probability that we correctly conclude that the average annual expenditure in the second health plan is smaller than that of the first plan when it really is smaller). If the critical value is decreased (moved to the left), that is, if we require stronger evidence to reject the null, the probability that we commit a Type I error decreases. However, our power also decreases. On the other hand, if we try to increase our power, the probability that we commit a Type I error increases. This figure shows the tradeoffs between Type I and Type II errors and power.

In this discussion, we considered only whether the second health plan's average annual expenditure is smaller than that of the first health plan and thus conducted a one-sided test. A two-sided test allows us to detect differences that are in the opposite direction from what was hypothesized (i.e., annual expenditures in Plan 2 are smaller or larger than in Plan 1). In that case, we would have both lower and upper critical values, which corresponds to our placing 2.5 percent in either "tail" of the null distribution. The lower critical value in Figure 6.2 would decrease as we would have only 2.5 percent rather than 5 percent probability in that tail, and the test would thereby require stronger evidence for rejection of the null. Generally, a two-sided test is conducted, as this strategy is more conservative than a one-sided approach and, if we reject based on such a test, we have very strong evidence against the null.

Types of Test Statistics. The type of hypothesis test used depends on the type of variable, or variables, being tested. Common tests for continuous quantitative variables such as age are

- The t-test for a single sample population mean;

- The t-test for comparing two different population means;

- The t-test for paired samples; and

- Analysis of variance tests (F-tests) for comparing several different population means.

T-tests take into account the fact that we do not usually know the true value of the standard deviation. If we do know the standard deviation, or if the sample size is large enough (at least 30 is a good rule of thumb) so that our uncertainty about the standard deviation no longer matters, a t-test is equivalent to a Normal or Z-test. Regardless of the type of test, all statistical hypothesis tests include a significance level (α), the probability of a Type II error (β), and a null hypothesis (H_0) and are conducted in the same manner as described above.

If our variable is qualitative rather than quantitative, other tests are applicable. We can test a population proportion, such as whether the Pap smear rate for enrolled women in one health plan is significantly different from the national proportion. Such tests are called Binomial proportion tests. If we have more than a single proportion, for example, the Pap smear rates in more than one age group, we may display our data in a contingency table, such as shown in Table 6.19. For this type of data, a chi-squared test is applicable. The null hypothesis is that whether the woman receives a Pap smear is not associated with (is inde-pendent of) her age. The alternative hypothesis is that the two characteristics are associated.

H_0 = receipt of Pap smear is not related to a woman's age.

H_1 = receipt of Pap smear is related to a woman's age.

In conducting or interpreting any hypothesis test, understanding the null and alternative hypotheses is crucial. In this example, the p-value for the chi-square is less than 0.001 and we conclude that receiving a Pap smear is associated with age, because we reject the null hypothesis (our p-value is less than 0.05) of no correlation. Snedecor and Cochran (1980) give details on how a chi-squared statistic is calculated.

Several hypothesis-testing pitfalls are useful to keep in mind. More detail on these pitfalls can be found in Freedman et al. (1991). Returning to our blood pressure hypothesis test example, the first point is that if a hypothesis test

Table 6.19

Sample Contingency Table

Age	Received Pap Smear?	
	Yes	No
18–49	50%	50%
	125	125
50+	70%	30%
	175	75

NOTE: Chi-square = 20, p < 0.001; n = 500.

yields a significant result (e.g., the treatment significantly reduced blood pressure), this result may not be clinically or practically significant. If our sample size is large enough, we can conclude that a clinically insignificant drop in blood pressure is statistically significant. If our sample size is too small, we can conclude that a clinically significant drop in blood pressure is not statistically significant. The second point is that we should refrain from conducting multiple tests, as we may fool ourselves into concluding that a significant result exists by committing a Type I error. For example, if we conduct 20 tests at significance level of 5 percent, on average we will conclude that one test is significant even though the treatment has no effect. This erroneous conclusion has occurred because we have committed a Type I error 5 percent of the time; that is, we have concluded that there is a significant effect from treatment when there actually is no effect in one out of the 20 tests. The third point is that a hypothesis test does not establish causality—we know two groups are different but we do not know why.

Prediction

In many cases, we will want to predict the outcome (dependent variable) for a future observation based on the value of that observation's independent variables. For example, we may want to predict total annual expenditure for medical services by a person of a certain age, physical history, socioeconomic status, and other relevant factors. This statistical task answers the question, "What do we expect?" for the person in question. Using the annual expenditure we have observed for people with similar characteristics, we predict the expenditure for an individual. To predict, we need to determine the relationship between the independent variables and the dependent variable. For example, are expenditures higher for older people than for younger people? What effect does socioeconomic status have on the level of expenditures? This relationship is known as a statistical model and may take many mathematical forms, depending on the variables used and the statistical assumptions made about the sampling situation and other details. We will never know how to predict perfectly the dependent variable, as we cannot measure every independent variable that might affect a person's annual expenditure for medical services. Thus, statistical models contain an error component (ε_i). The effect of this error term is uncertain and is estimated using probability.

The most common type of mathematical relationship to use is a linear one, and the resulting model is called a *linear regression*. For the annual expenditure example, we might write the model as:

$$\text{Annual expenditures for person i} = \beta_0 + \beta_1(\text{age})_i + \varepsilon_i$$

In this example, our outcome (dependent variable) is the annual expenditure for each person. The independent variable is the person's age. The outcome is related to the independent variable via a linear relationship, which is a good approximation of the true relationship in many situations.

The βs are called the *regression coefficients* and tell us the direction and magnitude of the effect each independent variable (or covariate) has on the outcome. For example, if the coefficient for age (β_1) is 5 and annual expenditures are measured in dollars, this means that for each additional year of age, a person on average spends an additional \$5 on medical services annually. β_0 is called the intercept and is the fixed value of the outcome variable that does not vary with different characteristics.

Usually, a simple linear regression is inadequate to represent the variety of factors that affect the outcome of interest. Thus, a *multiple linear regression* is more frequently used. The name reflects that the coefficients in the model are linear and more than one independent variable is included. We can write a generic multiple linear regression model using mathematical notation:

$$Y_i = \beta_0 + \beta_1 x_{1i} + \beta_2 x_{2i} + \ldots \beta_p x_{pi} + \varepsilon_i$$

where

$$Y = \text{dependent variable,}$$

$$(x_1, x_2, \ldots, x_p) = \text{independent variables,}$$

$$\beta_j = \text{coefficient for independent variable } j \text{ (effect of } x_j \text{ on Y),}$$

$$\varepsilon = \text{error term, and}$$

$$i = \text{individual } i.$$

In some situations, we are interested in the effect of a specific independent variable or set of variables on the dependent variable, but we want to ensure that the effects of other independent variables are eliminated. The terminology generally used to describe this type of analysis is that we will "control for potential confounding factors." The model allows us to see the unique contribution that each independent variable makes to predicting the outcome. We can determine if the effects of the independent variables are statistically significant using the same general testing approach described above under hypothesis testing.

A variety of multivariate models may be used, with the preferred technique dependent on the types of variables in the model and the question that is being answered. Table 6.20 shows the different types of models used for different combinations of dependent and independent variables.

The following section provides a sampler of different modeling techniques to acquaint you with some possible approaches. You should consult statistical and content experts to determine the optimal technique for any given problem.

Multiple Linear Regression Models. We begin with another example of multiple linear regression, which is used when the dependent variable is a continuous variable. For example, say that you want to estimate the proportion of people in a county that are uninsured as a function of the characteristics of that county. (This example is taken from Diehr et al., 1991). Using the notation from the generic expression for this type of model, let

Y = percentage of residents who are uninsured,

x_1 = per capita income,

x_2 = percentage unemployed, and

x_3 = percentage on welfare.

So, the model might look like this:

$$\% \text{ uninsured in county } i = \beta_0 + \beta_1 (\text{per capita income})_i$$
$$+ \beta_2 (\% \text{ unemployed})_i + \beta_3 (\% \text{ welfare})_i + \varepsilon_i$$

Table 6.20

Common Analytic Techniques

Dependent Variable	Independent Variable	Analytic Technique
Continuous (annual expenditure)	Continuous (age)	Multiple linear regression
Continuous (annual expenditure)	Categorical (gender)	Regression analysis of variance (ANOVA)
Continuous (annual expenditure)	Continuous and categorical (age and gender)	Regression analysis of co-variance (ANOCOVA)
Categorical (immunization source: health plan, school, public health clinic)	Categorical (insured or not insured)	Contingency table analysis Log-linear models
Binary (immunized or not)	Continuous or categorical (age, insurance status)	Multiple logistic regression

SOURCE: Adapted from Dobson (1990).

Once the model is estimated using statistical software, the results might look like this:

$$\text{Predicted \% uninsured in county } i = 4.0 - 0.0001(\text{per capita income})_i$$
$$+ 1.5(\text{\% unemployed})_i + 0.2(\text{\% welfare})_i$$

The number in front of each independent variable in this equation is the estimated effect of that variable on the proportion uninsured, holding all other factors constant. With these results, you could predict the proportion of uninsured in an area if you had information on the other variables in the equation. If the average per capita income in a county was $10,000, the unemployment rate was 9 percent, and the proportion of the population on welfare was 5 percent, you would predict the proportion of uninsured by substituting this information into the equation:

$$\text{Predicted \% uninsured} = 4.0 - 0.0001(\$10,000) + 1.5(9\%) + 0.2(5\%)$$
$$= 17.5\%$$

This analysis allows you to predict how the proportion of uninsured persons changes as each independent variable in the equation changes. For example:

- For every $1,000 increase in per capita income, the proportion of uninsured decreases one-tenth of one percentage point. The negative sign in front of the regression coefficient indicates that the dependent variable decreases as the independent variable increases.

- A one percentage point increase in the unemployment rate will increase the proportion of uninsured by 1.5 percentage points.

- A one percentage point increase in the percentage of the population on welfare will cause the proportion of the population that is uninsured to increase by two-tenths of a percentage point.

This is a simplified example intended to give a general sense of the type of analysis done with multiple regression and an idea of how the results might be used to generate information.

Multiple linear regression analysis is appropriate when several independent variables are likely to simultaneously affect the dependent variable and when the dependent variable is a qualitative or continuous variable.

We have ignored here a variety of technical issues that are needed to interpret the results. For example, we have not discussed how we use theoretical or empirical evidence to determine which independent variables should be in our model or the assumptions that underlie the model. Nor have we discussed the precision of our regression coefficients or predictions. In fact, we can test the significance of our coefficients. For example, does the percentage on welfare really affect the percentage of uninsured or is the observed positive effect just due to chance (i.e., to the particular sample chosen)? In addition, we must remember that our results are based on the data we have available. Whether the model and the results will be the same or similar if different data are used is an important test of how well the model is likely to perform in subsequent use. One technique that is frequently used is "split half" cross-validation. This procedure fits the model using a random half of the data set (i.e., the independent variables are chosen and their regression coefficients are estimated); once a final model is selected, the model is run on the second half of the data to see how well it predicts the outcome for those observations. This is a commonly used validation strategy, but it requires sufficient sample size to split the data in half. In any event, testing the sensitivity of the model by varying the underlying assumptions and data is an important part of the model validation process.

Analysis of Variance. ANOVA is a subset of regression and is used to examine how much of the variation in a dependent continuous variable is explained by qualitative (categorical) independent variables. The simplest type of ANOVA model is one that involves a single independent variable; it is known as a one-way ANOVA. The independent variable is often called a factor in such a model. The ANOVA technique can be used to compare the mean values of subgroups defined by the factor to determine whether they differ from one another. For example, if the dependent variable is blood pressure and the factor is ethnicity (white, black, Asian, and Hispanic), the one-way ANOVA allows simultaneous comparison of the average blood pressure for whites, the average blood pressure for blacks, the average blood pressure for Asians, and the average blood pressure for Hispanics. More complicated ANOVA models include two factors (a two-way ANOVA) or more.

Essentially, ANOVA compares the amount of the variance in the dependent variable that is explained by the independent variables to the amount of variance that is explained by chance alone. The statistic used to compare the two amounts of variance is the *F-statistic.* If this statistic is large, the independent variables explain a relatively large portion of the variability in the dependent variable. In our previous example, a large F-statistic means that the variation across people in blood pressure can be well-explained by ethnicity. A statistical hypothesis test is conducted to determine if the F-statistic is large enough to imply a strong relationship between blood pressure and ethnicity. If the F-statistic is large enough, we reject the null hypothesis that the average blood pressures in the four ethnic groups are equal.

ANOVA is appropriate when the independent variables are qualitative and the dependent variable is continuous.

Analysis of Covariance. ANOCOVA combines standard linear regression analysis and ANOVA. The dependent variable is continuous and the independent variables are either continuous or qualitative. This is a fairly common technique, as there are many instances in which combining types of independent variables in the analysis provides the best method for modeling the outcome of interest. In our previous example, we may be interested in determining the relationship between the blood pressure outcome and two independent variables: ethnicity (qualitative) and age (continuous).

ANOCOVA is appropriate when the independent variables are qualitative and continuous and the dependent variable is continuous.

Multiple Logistic Regression. This technique is conceptually similar to multiple linear regression and is used when the dependent variable is binary (i.e., it can take on only two values—the child was immunized or not). The approach may be expanded to apply to polytomous—or many—outcomes (i.e., it can take on multiple, discrete values, such as (1) has no insurance, (2) belongs to a fee-for-service plan, or (3) belongs to an HMO) as well, though we will not discuss that extension here.

In logistic regression, the independent variables can be either continuous or categorical. When logistic regression is used, the results are frequently presented as *odds ratios,* which is a way of expressing the relative effect of the independent variable on the dependent variable. The odds ratio is useful because it puts all factors onto a common scale—the effects of each independent variable in the model can be directly compared holding the values of all other variables in the model constant. The general interpretation of odds ratios is as follows. If the odds ratio for a particular independent variable is greater than one, this indicates that the odds that the dependent variable occurs increase with higher values of the independent variable. If the odds ratio for a particular independent variable is less than one, this indicates that the odds that the dependent variable occurs decrease with higher values of the independent variable. Thus, if the outcome is whether the respondent smokes, an odds ratio of two for the independent variable age means that for every additional year of age, a respondent has twice the odds of smoking.

Multiple logistic regression is appropriate when the independent variables are qualitative or continuous and the dependent variable is binary.

For example, in a study conducted in Los Angeles County, several independent variables were found to be important factors associated with immunization status for Hispanic children (Table 6.21). For each additional child in the

Table 6.21

Sample Logistic Regression Results

Dependent Variable: Were a child's immunizations age-appropriate at 12 months?		
Independent Variable	Odds Ratio	P-Value
General characteristics		
No. of children in household	0.75	$p < 0.05$
Respondent working full/part-time	1.71	$p < 0.05$
Education of respondent	1.06	$p < 0.05$
Belief shots any time are ok	1.16	$p < 0.05$
Belief shots prevent colds/diarrhea	0.78	$p < 0.05$
Personal resources		
No. of barriers to getting shots	0.86	$p < 0.10$
System contact/access		
Inadequate prenatal care	0.38	$p < 0.01$
Well-child care from private doctor	1.69	$p < 0.05$

household, the odds of a child getting immunized are 75 percent. That is, a child from a household with a greater number of children was less likely to get immunized. The odds of immunization for a child in a household where the respondent parent worked outside of the home are 1.71 times the odds for a child in a household where the respondent parent did not work outside the home. Table 6.21 shows only the independent variables that were statistically significant in the model, so all p-values are less than 5 percent.

Because this is a multivariate model, we can see the individual effect of each independent variable on the outcome when all other variables in the model are held constant. This helps us to understand the relative importance of each variable in the model. In this case, we can see that respondents working outside the home and receiving well-child care from a private doctor are the most powerful variables associated with a child having appropriate immunizations by age one, since these two independent variables have the largest odds ratios. We can also identify risk factors for not getting immunized such as inadequate prenatal care.

Time Series Analysis. Time series analysis is a special technique used to make predictions. The models described previously are referred to as structural models because they make predictions about the future values of a dependent variable based on its relationship to a set of independent variables. In some situations, however, such structural models are either not useful (e.g., the errors in the predictions are too large) or not feasible (e.g., we do not understand the structure of the relationship between the dependent variable and the independent variables). Time series models track prior changes in the outcome over time and use the past pattern of behavior to predict future movements in the dependent variable (Pindyck and Rubinfeld, 1991). Time series models are often used for economic or business forecasting. Three common types of time series analyses are used in health policy analysis:

- **Trend analysis** typically models a linear change in a dependent variable over time. Tracking the growth in health expenditures is an example of a trend analysis.

- **Seasonal patterns** are used to model phenomena that fluctuate with the seasons. Many disease patterns, such as colds and flu, exhibit seasonal patterns and understanding the nature of the fluctuation as a function of time may be useful for a variety of purposes. For example, knowing when to target administration of influenza vaccines requires understanding the seasonal pattern of this disease. For certain studies, understanding fluctuations in symptoms that result from changes in the seasons can affect sampling decisions; conditions such as asthma are often exacerbated by increased pollen levels during spring months and this may mean that asthmatics studied during those months will appear more severely affected than asthmatics studied at different time periods.

- **Random patterns** (i.e., stochastic) are perhaps one of the most common reasons for conducting time series analysis—because a relationship between values of the dependent variable can be observed over time but are not explained by any set of independent variables.

Choosing the correct time series model depends on the purpose of the analysis and the nature of the data available. Consulting an expert in forecasting and other time series techniques is essential for ensuring proper application of the technique. Time series analysis often requires more assumptions than regression and the results may be particularly sensitive to those assumptions, which consequently must be carefully evaluated. For an example of time series analysis combined with regression analysis, see Mitchell (1993), who examines time trends in inpatient physician spending. By analyzing the time trends in spending and then modeling possible explanations for these trends, she concludes that controls over both technology and the number of physicians caring for a patient in the hospital are necessary for constraining the rate of growth in physician inpatient expenditures.

Decision Analysis. Decision analysis is a method used to compare alternative strategies (e.g., whether to have surgery) by structuring the decision in a way that takes into account both the preferences of the individual making the choice and the probabilities of certain outcomes from each of the possible choices. Many methods for making patients more active participants in decisions about their health care involve decision analytic techniques. A simple example (from Behn and Vaupel, 1982) will illustrate the basic approach. They begin by describing the decision problem in prose:

Mr. Watt has two alternatives.

- Option 1: not to have bypass surgery. The result of this choice is certain. Mr. Watt will continue to live (for the next 10 years) but will also continue to have chest pain (angina).

- Option 2: to have bypass surgery. There are two possible outcomes of this choice. There is a 90 percent chance that the operation will be a success; Mr. Watt will live for 10 years and will have no angina. There is, however, a 10 percent chance that Mr. Watt will die during surgery.

Based on this description, the decision tree can be drawn as shown in Figure 6.3.

The decision tree contains the same information as presented above verbally, but it may be a more helpful tool for decisionmaking. The authors point out several advantages to the use of decision trees: (1) Drawing the decision tree requires separating the problem into manageable parts, (2) the decision is explicitly simplified through the choice of which components to include in the decision tree, (3) an individual's beliefs about uncertainty and preferences for different outcomes can be specified, and (4) the decision nodes are organized in the proper sequence.

To complete the decision analysis shown in Figure 6.3, we would have to assign values to the three terminal events in the tree: "Live, but with angina," "Live without angina," and "Die." Such an assignment is difficult given the nature of these events; techniques such as time tradeoff and standard gamble are used to assign values for these events. Given the estimated values, you can calculate the expected value (the weighted average of the values where the weights are

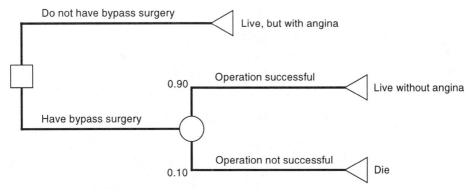

Figure 6.3—A Decision Tree for Bypass Surgery

the probabilities) for each decision and choose the decision that has the maximum value. For example, the "Do not have bypass surgery" decision choice has an expected value equal to the value of the event "Live, but with angina." The "Have bypass surgery" decision choice has an expected value equal to 0.90 times the value of the event "Live without angina" plus 0.10 times the value of the event "Die." Whichever decision choice has a larger expected value is chosen.

An example of an application of this analysis technique can be found in Oddone et al. (1993), a study that assessed the cost-effectiveness of the hepatitis B vaccine for predialysis patients. The researchers concluded that although additional cases of hepatitis B could be prevented through the immunization of predialysis patients, the costs are high and the decision should be determined by examining the local prevalence of hepatitis B. To be cost-effective, the incidence of the infection would have to increase from 0.6 to 38 percent.

Cost-Benefit or Cost-Effectiveness Analysis. Cost-benefit analysis is a method for making decisions between competing choices for public expenditures (Warner and Luce, 1982). The rationale for cost-benefit analysis is that economic efficiency should govern choices about the use of resources. The basic approach (from Stokey and Zeckhauser, 1978) is

1. Identify all potential projects competing for the same resources (e.g., vaccinating all children under age two, or increasing screening mammography among women over age 50).

2. Determine all of the favorable and unfavorable effects on society (both now and in the future) associated with implementing these projects (e.g., reductions in morbidity and mortality, increased identification of persons with disease, or increased number of reactions to vaccine).

3. Assign dollar values to each of these effects; favorable effects are classified as benefits and unfavorable effects are classified as costs. Because the problem is one of comparing different types of projects, the benefits and costs are generally monetized, that is, some dollar value is placed on them.

4. Calculate the net benefit (total benefit minus total cost or total benefit divided by total cost).

5. Select among the alternatives. The analytic technique implies that you select the project or set of projects that confers the greatest benefit on society within the budget that is available.

Cost-benefit analysis is difficult to use in many complex health policy problems because there is no consensus on how to assign a monetary value to various outcomes (e.g., the dollar value of a year of life saved). There have been continuing debates about how to value outcomes such as death or disability, the additional years of life provided by a medical treatment, and so on. When conducting any analysis, the assumptions made should be clearly stated and the sensitivity of the results to the assumption choices should be evaluated.

A related approach is cost-effectiveness analysis, which is used when you are comparing different methods for achieving the same outcome. For example, if you are interested in whether medical therapy or surgery is more cost-effective, you could use cost-effectiveness analysis to make that determination. An example of an application of this technique can be found in Wagner et al. (1991) examining the cost-effectiveness of colorectal cancer screening in the elderly. They compared four strategies for periodically screening persons age 65–85 for colorectal cancer and examined the costs (i.e., health care expenditures) and effects (i.e., life expectancy) of each strategy. They concluded that although colorectal cancer screening is costly, the medical benefits to the elderly are justifiable from a cost-effectiveness perspective.

A host of analytic techniques are available. To assist you with learning more about the techniques discussed above as well as others, see the references in Table 6.22.

INTERPRETING THE RESULTS

Having completed the analysis, you must now think about the results of your analysis to decide what actions to take or not take.

The first step is to assess whether the results make sense. You should evaluate the results in the context of what people have found in prior studies and what appears to occur in the real world. For example, if you were to find that the likelihood of having insurance coverage declined as income increased, this result would be inconsistent with prior research studies and what we tend to observe in the world. You should always think about whether results make sense and, if they do not, what could account for the different finding. In some cases, the finding may, in fact, be real. In other cases, the results may be due to model misspecification (e.g., omitted variable) or data problems. It is very important to check all possible reasons your results differ from what others have found or are counterintuitive. There may be good explanations, but you need to be prepared to explain the difference.

The second step in interpretation is deciding if your result is statistically significant or meaningful. This involves computing a test (discussed above) to assess whether the result is due to a real effect (the treatment has an effect) as opposed to chance. Note that even if your result is not statistically significant, your results may be practically important.

Table 6.22

List of Suggested References for Conducting Analyses

Reference	Analysis Topics Covered
Basic books	
Stokey and Zeckhauser (1978)	Cost-benefit analysis, simulation, discounting, linear programming, decision analysis, queuing models
Mausner and Kramer (1985)	Epidemiology, study design
Freedman et al. (1991)	Descriptive statistics, regression, correlation, probability theory, sampling, tests of significance
Mansfield (1991)	Descriptive statistics, probability sampling, sampling designs, hypothesis testing, statistical estimation, regression
Bailar and Mosteller (1992)	Use of statistics in medical studies, emphasis on interpretation
Multivariate modeling (logistic and linear)	
Chatfield and Collins (1980)	Multivariate analysis, etc. (same as Johnson and Wichern, 1998)
Draper and Smith (1981)	Multiple regression
Weisberg (1985)	Multiple regression
Johnson and Wichern (1988)	Multivariate statistical models—principal components, factor analysis, canonical correlation analysis, discriminate analysis, clustering
Hosmer and Lemeshow (1989)	Logistic regression
Neter et al. (1990)	Multiple regression, ANOVA, experimental design
Multivariate techniques	
Chatfield and Collins (1980)	Multivariate analysis, etc. (same as Johnson and Wichern, 1988)
Johnson and Wichern (1988)	Multivariate statistical models—principal components, factor analysis, canonical correlation analysis, discriminate analysis, clustering
Sampling	
Cochran (1977)	Simple random sampling, estimating sample size, stratified random sampling, cluster sampling, sources of error in surveys
Levy and Lemeshow (1991)	Simple random sampling, etc. (same as Cochran, 1977)
Kish (1965)	Simple random sampling, etc. (same as Cochran, 1977)
Special topics—statistics	
Fleiss (1981)	Significance tests for proportions and rates, contingency tables
Miller (1981)	Survival analysis, life-table analysis
Chatfield (1989)	Time series, ARIMA and state-space models
Petitti (1994)	Cost-effectiveness, decision analysis, and meta-analysis
Yin (1994)	Case study analysis
Special topics—economics and cost analysis	
Warner and Luce (1982)	Cost-benefit and cost-effectiveness analysis
Koutsoyiannis (1985)	Regression, analysis of variance, simultaneous equation models, lagged variables
Pindyck and Rubinfeld (1991)	Regression models, multi-equation simulation models, time series models

The third step is to assess whether the result is important, either clinically or from a practical standpoint (i.e., practically significant, regardless of whether or not statistically significant). This is determined by looking at the size of the effect or the size of the coefficient in a model. There is no absolute rule for making this determination: You will need to gauge the importance in the context of your specific problem. For example, a very small reduction in likelihood of using services by the Medicare population that could be achieved by changing patient cost-sharing requirements might still have a very large effect on total program expenditures. This is because of the size of the population that would be affected by this change. In contrast, a very large change may not be important if it affects relatively few people. For example, instituting patient cost-sharing for a very rare illness may have limited effect because few people will be affected by the provision, even if cost-sharing is shown to lower use among those persons with the health condition. In evaluating the practical significance of your study results, you should ask yourself, "What difference would it make if I acted on this result?" By answering this question you can avoid wasting valuable resources on something with low payoff potential.

The fourth step is to assess what should be done next, judging by your study results. As a result of the study you may conclude that you need (1) to further analyze your data, (2) to examine a new question identified through your analysis, (3) to implement a policy change and monitor the effect of the change, and (4) to reevaluate the same question in the future to see whether things have changed and, if so, in what direction.

To summarize, the last stage of any analysis should address the following questions:

- Do the results make sense?
- Are the results "real" or simply due to chance?
- If the results make sense and are real, are they meaningful?
- What should be done next?

Chapter Seven

DEVELOPING AND USING A CLINICAL INFORMATION SYSTEM

by Eve A. Kerr, Elizabeth A. McGlynn, and Cheryl Damberg

INTRODUCTION

This chapter highlights the key issues that must be addressed in constructing integrated clinical information systems. Clinical data allow analysts to evaluate the process, outcomes, and costs of medical care at various levels (e.g., provider, hospital, clinic, health plan, or employer group). Although you could currently answer specific questions by collecting data from a variety of independent sources, in practice such a data collection effort is time-consuming and expensive and in some cases may yield inaccurate results (for example, using administrative data to determine diagnosis or comorbidity). An integrated clinical information system would significantly enhance analytic opportunities. Elements of such a data base are listed in Table 7.1.

The decision about what information to collect should be based on the need to answer specific questions. These questions could address a variety of topics, including quality of care, access to care, costs of treatment, and the health of a population. Examples of such questions include

Table 7.1

Elements of a Clinical Data Base

Original Data Source	Examples of Available Information
Enrollment files	Age, income, race/ethnicity
Administrative files	Type of visits, tests ordered
Medical records	Treatments, severity of illness
Laboratory data	Results of tests
Pharmaceutical data	Medication prescribed
Radiologic and other procedure data	Results of procedures
Birth certificates	Prenatal care, birthweight
Death certificates	Cause, time, and place of death
Facility files	Availability of services, hours of operation
Patient surveys	Functional status

- How do the quality of care delivered and the costs of care differ across providers for patients with a specific clinical condition?

- How appropriate is the use of a specific surgical procedure among health plans?

- How do changes in reimbursement policies for preventive services affect rates of use?

As mentioned, if one were currently trying to answer such questions, it would be necessary to draw data from a variety of existing sources delineated in Table 7.1. Currently, each of these data sources has limitations that affect the reliability of evaluations (see Chapter Five). Further, lack of integration and unique patient and provider identifiers makes the evaluation of quality and clinical outcomes cumbersome. In contrast, an integrated data base that contains essential elements necessary to answer specific questions would facilitate answering a variety of questions. Such an integrated system would depend on accurate data that are prospectively collected, allowing for valid and efficient analysis and unique identifiers for patients, providers, and facilities. Focused medical record review, automated entry of key clinical sources, or specific surveys could provide additional data, if necessary. If a specific piece of information does not help answer the questions likely to be posed, either directly or indirectly (e.g., for use as a covariate in severity adjustment), the benefit of collecting the data element may not outweigh the expense. In this chapter, we will outline issues to consider in collecting clinical data.

HOW WILL A CLINICAL INFORMATION SYSTEM WORK?

A clinical information system incorporates various aspects of clinical data into an integrated whole. Pryor et al. (1985) stated that "a clinical data base is created when well-defined, discrete, and continuous data elements concerning patients are routinely recorded and coupled with outcome descriptors." Data from a variety of sources could be captured in real-time and entered into an electronic data base accessible to analysts. For example, to assess quality of care for diabetes in a health plan, the clinical data base would capture information on patient demographics from enrollment data, type of patient visits from administrative data, level of glycemic control from medical record data, and quality of life from focused patient surveys. Until these data bases become more widely available, analysts must obtain the data from original sources (e.g., administrative, medical record, or patient survey). A clinical information system would allow the analyst to answer specific questions more accurately and efficiently.

HOW DO CLINICAL DATA DIFFER FROM ADMINISTRATIVE DATA?

Administrative data have been used to examine variations in hospitalization rates, appropriateness, and quality of care (Roos et al., 1990; Hannan et al., 1992b). You may think that it is sufficient to use only administrative data in evaluating utilization, quality, access, and costs. However, as detailed in Chapter Five, administrative data have several important limitations (see Table 7.2). Administrative data may not contain accurate diagnostic information; may confuse comorbidity with complications; may lack information on clinical risk factors, health status, and process of care; and may be difficult to evaluate longitudinally. These limitations have important implications in the evaluation of clinical conditions. For example, Hannan et al. (1992b) found that clinical data were better able to predict in-hospital mortality from CABG surgery than administrative data. In addition, clinical data are better suited for evaluation of medical care in the outpatient setting, where accurate diagnoses and severity adjustment from administrative data present an even greater challenge. Integration of accurate and detailed clinical information with relevant encounter-level data in a clinical data base makes valid interpretation possible.

Until a functional information system is operational, you could still use administrative data (coupled with accurate enrollment data) to answer questions for which severity adjustment is not required. For example, if you want to investigate whether screening mammography rates differ from one health plan to another, it is probably sufficient to use procedure codes as long as the coding system is consistent across plans (i.e., screening mammography is coded the same in all plans) and you have accurate enrollment data (i.e., the eligible population for the indicator, such as women age 50 and older, can be identified). Roos et al. (1990) have shown that using administrative data alone may be sufficient to answer certain questions, such as differences in utilization across medical market areas, because you can generally estimate the population in a market area. However, if you want to assess the rate of cerebrovascular accidents (CVAs or strokes) in patients with hypertension, collecting clinical data is crucial. Clinical data supply detailed longitudinal information about hypertension control, comorbidities, and severity of CVAs, which allows for accurate severity adjustment.

Table 7.2

Advantages of Clinical over Administrative Data

Clinical Data	Administrative Data
Cover entire enrolled population	Cover only users of health care
More accurate for severity adjustment	Limited for severity adjustment
More accurate clinical diagnosis	Diagnoses subject to coding errors
Allow assessment of process of care	Content of care processes limited

WHY IS SEVERITY ADJUSTMENT IMPORTANT?

According to Iezzoni (1997), the goal of severity adjustment is "to account for pertinent patient characteristics before making inferences about the effectiveness of care." Why is this important? Generally speaking, patients who are sicker at baseline (i.e., their main condition is more serious or they have other coexisting health conditions upon admission to the hospital) may be expected to have poorer outcomes than healthier patients, despite appropriate medical care. If a hospital, provider, or health plan has attracted a larger proportion of sicker patients, their outcomes may appear worse despite identical process of care. For example, when the Health Care Financing Administration (HCFA) initially released hospital-level mortality figures in 1986, they failed to adequately adjust for differences in patients' severity of illness (Iezzoni, 1997). HCFA reported that 142 hospitals had significantly higher death rates than predicted and 127 had lower rates. The facility with the highest death rate was a hospice caring for terminally ill patients, which you would expect to have a high death rate. Adequate adjustment for the patients' severity of illness should have captured these patients' risk of death and adjusted for it in the model, thus leveling the playing field to permit fair comparisons.

Lack of adequate severity adjustment can yield false estimates and may have serious consequences for hospitals, health plans, and providers. New York State publishes data on mortality after coronary artery bypass graft (CABG) surgery by hospital and provider. Their reports are based on a detailed discharge document that physicians and hospitals must complete for each patient undergoing CABG. These documents include extensive questions on factors known to influence mortality after CABG (e.g., cardiac status and comorbidities), and these elements are used for severity adjustment. This type of data collection is an example of clinical data reporting not generally available from hospital discharge data or encounter data. However, a clinical information system could routinely collect this type of data. Because of such careful severity adjustment, there are many fewer questions about the validity of these reports (Hannan et al., 1990). Severity adjustment is addressed in greater detail in Chapter Nine.

WHAT ARE THE CHARACTERISTICS OF AN IDEAL CLINICAL INFORMATION SYSTEM?

In general, an integrated clinical information system should facilitate answering clinically detailed questions posed by a variety of stakeholders. We will consider several attributes that contribute to an ideal clinical information system; these are summarized in Table 7.3.

Table 7.3

Attributes of an Ideal Clinical Data Base

Issue	Importance
Valid diagnoses	Provides accuracy in drawing conclusions
Uniform data	Facilitates comparisons
Severity adjustment	Adjusts outcomes for baseline patient differences; facilitates comparisons
Real-time data collection	Allows for prompt analysis
Unique identifiers	Allows for analyses across different types of files
Comprehensive data	Expands analytic opportunities and problem-solving capabilities

Diagnoses Must Be Valid

A clinical information system should contain valid diagnoses. This is important to ascertain that analyses are done for the true conditions of interest and that differences among patients can be taken into account, thus yielding accurate conclusions. Comorbidities are diagnoses that coexist with the principal diagnosis (or diagnosis of interest) but are unrelated in etiology or causality to the principal diagnosis (Iezzoni, 1997). For example, a patient whose main diagnosis is coronary artery disease (because he is in the hospital to receive CABG surgery) may also have comorbidities of asthma and rheumatoid arthritis. Currently, diagnoses for visits and hospitalizations are coded on administrative forms primarily for reimbursement considerations. Therefore, when there is some flexibility (e.g., the doctor lists more than one diagnosis or the severity of a given condition is not clear), the person filling out the charge or encounter documents may list first (as principal diagnosis) the diagnosis most likely to generate the highest level of reimbursement.

You can see that this may yield inaccurate diagnoses. How can a clinical information system improve this situation?

- Administrative data should be integrated with clinical data, so that it will be difficult to request reimbursement for a diagnosis that the clinical data do not substantiate.

- Outside parties (e.g., payors) can more easily verify the diagnoses by reviewing clinical data.

- Diagnoses can be entered automatically from physician notes.

Instead of discarding the current method of coding diagnoses (e.g., ICD-9 codes), however, it is preferable to add to the current structure of listing diagnoses and comorbidities. The current coding scheme does not differentiate between complications, or sequelae of the principal diagnosis, and comorbidities

(Hannan et al., 1992b). For example, the patient receiving CABG surgery for coronary artery disease may develop pneumonia after surgery. This is a complication of surgery, whereas pneumonia suffered before surgery would have been a comorbidity that might increase the risk of poor outcomes from surgery. An extra digit or letter added to the ICD-9-CM codes for pneumonia would allow you to make this distinction. In addition, clinical criteria should be developed for using specific diagnostic codes. Hospital diagnoses may still be based on ICD-9 codes, but these codes would be more precise than before.

Accurate classification of diagnoses and comorbidities is also important in ambulatory settings to evaluate practice patterns, process of care, and outcomes. Ambulatory diagnoses may be even less accurate than hospital diagnoses, in part because reimbursement has been linked to the length of the visit rather than to the specific diagnosis, except when a specific procedure is performed (e.g., skin biopsy). Since a clinical information system should contain the diagnosis reported by the physician, rather than being designed for reimbursement purposes, diagnostic validity should be enhanced. Ambulatory coding in a clinical data base may also take into account the reason for the visit (e.g., a symptom or care not related to illness), rather than a particular diagnosis.

Data Must Be Uniform and Consistent

To make comparisons regarding quality or costs, track the prevalence of a condition in a community, or understand how the practice patterns of a particular physician vary from those of another, you need to be sure that the data reported are consistent and uniform. For example, an employer may wish to compare the quality of care given to adults with congestive heart failure in different hospitals. However, patients with congestive heart failure may be listed under one of many diagnoses (e.g., congestive heart failure, viral cardiomyopathy, or ischemic cardiomyopathy) and providers may use different codes for patients with very similar clinical conditions because there has been no specific agreement on when the diagnosis of congestive heart failure should be assigned—i.e., for what set of symptoms, signs, or test results. Accordingly, Iezzoni and Moskowitz (1998) have shown that for the same clinical condition, patients in North Carolina were more likely to receive a diagnosis of coronary atherosclerosis, whereas New Jersey patients were more likely to receive a diagnosis of angina pectoris. To encourage uniformity in data coding, and thus to make more precise analyses possible, rules regarding diagnoses must be established and communicated to providers a priori. Further, a uniform system of coding, as detailed in Chapter Five, would allow you to identify all patients with the same diagnosis.

Diagnoses are only one area where uniformity is key. For example, developers and users of clinical information systems must agree on units for specific laboratory data and reported names for pharmaceutical data (i.e., generic versus trade) to efficiently make comparisons. Alternatively, computer programs could be written to convert disparate units or drug names to the agreed-upon units and names to be used in analyses. These changes should be made when the system is designed to make a clinical data base not only integrated but also uniform, useful, and efficient.

Data Must Allow for Severity or Risk Adjustment

The clinical information system also needs to contain data elements that allow for accurate severity adjustment. This is important because patients with similar diagnoses or undergoing similar procedures may experience different outcomes partly because they have different baseline risks. Differences in outcomes may result either from the severity of the disease for which treatment is sought (e.g., left main disease is a more severe form of heart disease than single vessel disease) or from comorbidities (e.g., if the patient with heart disease also had diabetes). For example, a 60-year-old man with chronic stable angina who is otherwise healthy may experience a better outcome from CABG surgery than another 60-year-old man with chronic stable angina, diabetes, chronic obstructive pulmonary disease, and renal insufficiency, despite identical processes of care. The second man has coexisting conditions or comorbidities that increase his risk of poor outcome. Similarly, a 50-year-old woman with poor heart functioning (e.g., ejection fraction < 35 percent) who undergoes CABG is at greater risk of dying than a 50-year-old woman whose heart works well (e.g., ejection fraction > 70 percent), because the severity of the first woman's condition is greater than that of the second woman. Our current system of coding does not allow for accurate assessment of severity and comorbidity. A clinical information system should capture information that would allow you to adjust for differences in severity and comorbidity when making comparisons regarding outcomes for providers, hospitals, and health plans. The principles of severity adjustment are detailed more fully in Chapter Nine.

Data Must Be Entered in "Real Time"

The data in a clinical information system should be collected at the time of the patient encounter to facilitate timely access to data. Prospective data collection offers several advantages. First, you can evaluate the process of care soon after it happened, which both more accurately reflects current practice and may allow for rapid cycle quality improvement. For example, an employer may wish to know how the costs and quality of one health plan compared with another before choosing which plan to offer to employees that year. If data are entered prospectively, the employer can get that information promptly and can react accordingly, instead of waiting 1-2 years, as may occur in the current system. Second, prospective data allow you to construct episodes of illness and follow care in a longitudinal fashion (i.e., consistent with guidelines). Finally, analyses based on prospective data collection may be subject to less bias than retrospective collection. If you retrospectively collect data for a particular purpose or with a specific hypothesis in mind, the purpose may influence the way data are collected; this might affect the accuracy of the data. In summary, prospective data allow analysts to

• Evaluate processes of care as they happen;

• Construct episodes of illness for clinical management; and

• Collect data in a less biased way.

The Information System Must Contain Unique Identifiers for Patients and Providers

Unique identifiers are an essential part of any information system being used for complex analyses. In fact, without unique identifiers, an integrated data base is not possible. A full discussion of unique identifiers can be found in Chapter Five.

Data Must Be Comprehensive

A clinical information system incorporates data from a variety of sources. Depending on the condition, these data could include information on

• Medical history;

• All diagnoses;

• Treatments;

• Response to treatment;

• Diagnostic procedures;

• Complications of procedures or treatment;

• Medication use;

• Follow-up plans;

• Laboratory tests;

• Pathology (e.g., results of Pap smears);

- Radiographic and imaging studies;

- Provider characteristics (e.g., specialty and training);

- Patient characteristics (e.g., race/ethnicity, gender, and income);

- Health status; and

- Quality of life.

Comprehensiveness is important because including and linking a wide range of care elements will allow accurate assessment of a variety of questions. Currently, data elements are in separate files and may be difficult to access and link. Some examples of specific data elements to collect for different conditions are more fully discussed at the end of this chapter.

Table 7.4 lists potential problems in a clinical data base and approaches to their solution.

USING CLINICAL DATA TO ADJUST FOR DIFFERENCES IN SEVERITY

The process of severity adjustment is a statistical method that allows you to make fair comparisons among different entities by accounting for baseline differences in patient characteristics. In other words, severity adjustment "corrects" for differences in patient characteristics or health risks that may influence the outcome of care, independent from medical treatment. As mentioned above, this includes both the severity of any single illness and the constellation of illnesses each patient has. You can then examine whether significant differences in outcomes are due to differences in the processes of care.

Using a clinical information system, you can account for many of the clinical differences between sicker and healthier patients. These clinical differences rest upon a variety of patient characteristics (e.g., comorbidity, age, and diagnosis). Several methods have been formulated to adjust for differences in severity of illness in hospital settings. According to Iezzoni (1997), who has detailed dimensions of severity and evaluated major severity-adjustment methods, several important dimensions of risk may affect outcomes, such as functional status, health status, comorbid conditions, and principal diagnosis. The key risk dimensions are listed in Chapter Nine.

It is probably not necessary to collect data on all of the key risk dimensions listed in Chapter Nine for each condition. However, certain dimensions will be crucial to all severity-adjustment analyses and should be collected routinely. These include age, gender, diagnoses, and severity of each diagnosis. One way to begin building clinical information systems is to select a few diagnoses on which to routinely collect detailed information. The clinical data base should

Table 7.4

Examples of Common Problems with Clinical Data and Proposed Solutions

Potential Problem	Solution
Lack of validity in diagnoses	Establish national detailed clinical criteria for common diagnoses and procedures Example—The diagnosis of congestive heart failure might be based on the following criteria: Signs and symptoms of intravascular and interstitial volume overload, including shortness of breath, rales, and edema; or Manifestations of inadequate tissue perfusion, such as fatigue or poor exercise tolerance; and Left ventricular ejection fraction of less than 40 percent (Konstam et al., 1994)
Lack of specificity in comorbidity coding	Request that NCHS and HCFA establish an additional digit on ICD-9-CM codes, which differentiates between complications and comorbidities
Lack of uniformity	Establish national detailed criteria for the most common diagnoses and procedures to be used in all sites Request that NCHS and HCFA expand ICD-9-CM codes to allow specific coding of procedures and tests (e.g., screening versus diagnostic mammogram) Health systems could ensure uniformity in coding either by using financial incentives to providers with spot checks to determine compliance, or by developing a program that allows a diagnosis to be used only if specific criteria are documented
Adjusting for differences in severity	Ensure that appropriate clinical data elements regarding severity and comorbidities are entered for specific target conditions Example—For each target condition, develop a set of questions about the condition and the severity-adjustment elements necessary to answer the questions; appropriate prompts in the computer program would ensure that severity-adjustment elements are entered whenever the target condition is coded
Delayed data entry and availability	Data need to be entered prospectively, integrated in real time, and made available promptly
Integrating different sources of data	Establish and use a unique identifier for enrollees, providers, and facilities
Lack of comprehensiveness	Ensure that the appropriate clinical data elements that allow questions about specific target conditions to be answered are entered in the data base Example—To evaluate processes of care for children with asthma, you need information on symptoms, physical exam, medication use, results of pulmonary function tests, and patient demographic characteristics; to also evaluate outcomes, data on health status and quality of life should be added

contain elements that allow accurate assessment on all of these dimensions. However, you must still decide which elements are essential to collect for specific conditions. For example, to assess severity of congestive heart failure, you may want the results of an echocardiogram, whereas for pneumonia, you may be more interested in the results of an arterial blood gas. Therefore, although there will be common elements for all conditions, specific data elements need to be identified to define severity for specific conditions. Some examples of severity-adjustment elements for specific conditions are found below. For a more detailed discussion of clinical severity-adjustment techniques, please see Chapter Nine.

WHAT ARE THE POTENTIAL USES OF A CLINICAL INFORMATION SYSTEM?

Clinical data have been used for technology assessment, studying efficiency of care, monitoring practice changes, evaluating compliance with screening recommendations, outcomes assessment, epidemiologic surveillance, prompts and reminders for providers, and education, among other functions (Pryor et al., 1985). You can pose and answer questions from a valid, uniform, and comprehensive data base in a number of different areas. Below, we identify various ways a clinical information system could be used.

Quality of Care

Main audiences: consumers, providers, health plans, employers, communities, and states.

In using the clinical information system to examine quality of care provided, an analyst would typically address questions related to the process, outcomes, and appropriateness of care. Examples of questions related to *process of care* include:

- What medications were prescribed for patients with coronary artery disease?

- Were specified screening tests obtained for patients with diabetes?

- What was the rate of mammography screening among women age 50 and older?

Examples of questions related to *outcomes* include:

- What complications arose at what rate for those undergoing coronary artery bypass graft surgery?

- How did patients' quality of life change after hip replacement?

- What proportion of patients with diabetes maintain their blood sugar at a normal level?

Questions regarding *appropriateness* might include:

- Among patients who received cholecystectomy in the previous year, what percentage of the operations were done for appropriate indications?

- Did everyone who could benefit from a coronary angiogram actually receive one?

All of these areas could be addressed from a variety of perspectives (e.g., employer, health plan, or state) and linkages between process and outcomes could be explored. A clinical information system allows you to accurately evaluate these questions because it contains the necessary clinical detail (i.e., laboratory test results, diagnostic findings, and comorbidities) for analysis.

Access to Care

Main audiences: consumers, health plans, communities, and states.

In evaluating access to care, you can examine whether all members of a population are obtaining the services from which they would benefit. For example:

- Do women of lower socioeconomic status (SES) obtain screening mammography at the same rate as women of higher SES?

- How do immunization rates of black children compare with those of white children?

- Are children from lower SES families hospitalized for asthma more frequently than children from higher SES families?

Data on race/ethnicity and SES should come from enhanced enrollment data. To answer many access questions accurately, you need to adjust the data for severity and comorbidities.

Costs and Cost-Effectiveness

Main audiences: health plans, employers, communities, and states.

A health plan may wish to compare the costs of coronary artery bypass graft surgery in two hospitals. Of course, the costs cannot be compared without a good method for severity adjustment because patients who are more severely ill may have differential expenses;[1] if two hospitals have different proportions of severely ill patients, this could affect their total or average costs of treatment. Measures of severity-adjusted costs may help health plans and employers make decisions about what hospitals, provider groups, and plans to contract with. Simply comparing costs, however, does not tell us anything about outcomes. To compare both the costs and the benefits of surgery in two hospitals, you need to perform a cost-effectiveness analysis. Cost-effectiveness analyses are especially important in the area of technology assessment but can be applied to a variety of situations. For example, an employer may find that one health plan is slightly more expensive than another for cardiac care, but that enrollees of that health plan with heart disease are more satisfied and have fewer sick days per year (after severity adjustment). A cost-effectiveness analysis may show that the benefit of the plan outweighs the additional costs (see Chapter Six).

Performance of Health Plans and Providers

Main audiences: consumers, providers, health plans, employers, and states.

An integrated clinical information system would allow health plans to efficiently produce profiles, or "report cards," of their performance (measures of quality, access, and cost) and to compare their performance to that of other plans. Since the results are adjusted for differences in the health risks of the population, more valid comparisons can be made using a clinical data base than was previously possible. Similarly, such analyses can be performed for individual providers if the number of patients with the condition being assessed is sufficiently large.

Effect of Public Health Programs

Main audiences: communities and states.

Public health programs are initiated to improve the health of populations. In *Healthy People 2000*, the U.S. Public Health Service (1990), for example, set goals for the nation in a number of important areas of health promotion and preventive services including (1) to increase the span of healthy life, (2) to reduce health disparities, and (3) to achieve access to preventive services.

To accomplish these goals, PHS set some specific targets in a variety of areas. Some examples include

---

[1]Care could be more expensive for patients whose severity contributes to longer lengths of stay or less expensive for those who die soon after admission for surgery.

- To reduce cigarette smoking to no more than 15 percent of adults;

- To reduce alcohol-related motor vehicle crash deaths to no more than 8.5 per 100,000 people (age adjusted); and

- To reduce disability from chronic conditions to no more than 8 percent of the population.

A statewide clinical information system would allow states to track whether they were being successful in meeting the national objectives. States may also initiate public health programs, such as a campaign to ensure that the vast majority of children under age two receive appropriate immunizations; these programs could be more readily evaluated with a statewide clinical information system.

Effect of Policy Changes on Health

Main audiences: health plans, employers, communities, and states.

In a similar way, you can evaluate the effect of policy changes on process and outcomes of care. For instance, a health plan may want to evaluate the effect of a new copayment (e.g., patient cost-sharing) on mammograms. The correct way to do this would be to either randomly assign some people to the copayment and compare mammogram rates for those with and without the copayment or to find a control group for comparison. A clinical information system would then allow the plan to assess how this policy change affects the rate at which screening mammograms are obtained and if it differentially affects mammography rates by income level or other enrollee characteristics.

Disease Surveillance

Main audiences: communities and states.

Knowing the number of persons with certain conditions (prevalence) may be important for a variety of reasons. For example, you can compare the prevalence of disease in two communities to identify areas with increased risk of disease, such as certain types of cancers that may be in part related to environmental factors (e.g., radiation). High prevalence of leukemia in a community, for example, might indicate the presence of an environmental hazard. Similarly, a clinical information system permits you to conduct other epidemiologic studies (such as prospective cohort studies and case-control studies) to evaluate the risk factors for various conditions. Tracking new cases (incidence) of particular infectious diseases may help indicate whether public health programs designed to prevent the transmission of communicable diseases are working.

Rate/Premium Setting

Main audiences: providers, health plans, and employers.

Some health plans or provider groups may attract sicker patients than other health plans, either by chance or as a result of the benefit package design or the costs of the plan. If all plans are reimbursed the same amount regardless of the health "risks" of the population they insure, such as occurs under community rating, the plan with higher-risk enrollees may be fiscally disadvantaged. Clinical data could be used to risk-adjust rates both prospectively and retrospectively (e.g., using baseline health status indicators) and by taking into account unexpected, large health expenditures by the population.

DECIDING WHAT CONDITIONS TO TARGET

How should designers of clinical information systems decide what areas to target for assessment? Rather than attempting to capture all clinical data elements for all possible conditions, we could more cost-effectively identify a subset of conditions for which data should be routinely collected and conduct special studies to answer other questions. For routine data collection, it is useful to think about conditions and procedures that are high volume, high cost, have a significant effect on health (i.e., morbidity and mortality), or for which care is believed to be highly variable or substandard. In addition, for quality of care analyses, you should target conditions for which medical interventions (i.e., improving appropriateness of coronary artery bypass graft surgery, increasing rates of mammography, or improving hypertensive control) result in improved health outcomes. Additionally, you may want to consider those clinical areas for which evidence-based practice guidelines have been developed. The target conditions may vary somewhat depending on the developers' perspective, although we would anticipate a large overlap for common areas. A health plan may be particularly interested in use of expensive services, an employer in conditions that cause loss of work days, and a state in communicable diseases. Clinical information systems have the potential to accommodate a variety of users.

To help system developers decide which conditions they may wish to target, we present a series of tables that list

- The most common chronic and acute conditions;

- The most frequent reasons for ambulatory visits, restricted activity days, and days lost from work for certain conditions; and

- High-volume and high-cost procedures.

It is important to note that a relatively small number of conditions account for the majority of mortality, morbidity, and costs in this country. Therefore, by focusing assessment of quality, access, and costs on these conditions, you will be able to have the greatest effect.

Common Conditions

Tables 7.5 and 7.6 identify the major causes of morbidity and mortality and the chronic conditions with the highest prevalence in the United States. Using the National Health Interview Survey (Collins, 1986), Siu et al. (1992) identified the major causes of mortality and morbidity (limited activity days) for five age groups: < 1, 1–17, 18–44, 45–64, and over 65.

Table 7.5

Major Causes of Morbidity and Mortality for Five Age Groups

Condition	Age Group
Infant mortality and related conditions	< 1
Otitis media	1–17
Asthma	1–17, 18–44
Accidents and injuries	1–17, 18–44, 45–64
Suicide	18–44
Acute respiratory conditions, including influenza	All ages
Breast cancer	18–44, 45–64
Coronary artery disease	18–44, 45–64, 65+
Arthritis	18–44, 45–64, 65+
Chronic bronchitis and emphysema	45–64, 65+
Colorectal cancer	45–64, 65+
Lung cancer	45–64, 65+
Stroke and cerebrovascular disease	45–64, 65+
Diabetes	45–64, 65+
Pneumonia	65+

SOURCE: Siu et al. (1992).

Limitations in Function

Table 7.7 lists the number of restricted activity days for selected chronic conditions. Restricted activity days are one way of measuring morbidity.

Table 7.8 lists acute conditions with high prevalence as well as the number of lost work days for those conditions for employees age 18 and over.

Table 7.6

Selected Chronic Conditions with Highest Prevalence in Rank Order, All Ages: United States, 1992

Condition	Prevalence (per 1,000 Persons)
1. Deformities and orthopedic impairments	140.6
2. Chronic sinusitis	135.6
3. Arthritis	127.8
4. High blood pressure	111.0
5. Hay fever or allergic rhinitis without asthma	96.7
6. Deafness and other hearing impairments	93.5
7. Heart disease	82.4
8. Chronic bronchitis	51.8
9. Asthma	46.2
10. Other headache (excludes tension headache)	41.3

SOURCE: CDC/National Center for Health Statistics (1997).

Table 7.7

Average Annual Number of Days of Restricted Activity from Selected Chronic Conditions, All Ages: United States, 1990–1992

Condition	Thousands of Days
Deformities or orthopedic impairments	599,569
Arthritis	445,381
Heart disease	399,680
Intervertebral disc disorders	187,530
High blood pressure	141,758
Diabetes	115,715
Cerebrovascular disease	118,046
Asthma	133,845

SOURCE: CDC/National Center for Health Statistics (1997).

Table 7.8

Number of Work-Loss Days from Selected Acute Conditions with Highest Incidence in Rank Order, All Ages: United States, 1994

Condition	Days Lost per 100 Currently Employed Persons Age 18 and Over
1. Respiratory conditions	105.3
Common cold	17.6
Influenza	56.4
Other acute respiratory infections	8.8
2. Injuries	115.5
3. Infective and parasitic diseases	21.6
4. Digestive system conditions	13.1

SOURCE: CDC/National Center for Health Statistics (1995).

Common Procedures

Another way to select clinical areas is to consider diseases for which medical procedures are commonly performed. Questions could include the appropriateness of procedures, their complication rate, costs and cost-effectiveness, and outcomes. The National Hospital Discharge Survey (CDC/NCHS, 1997b) has identified high-volume procedures and diagnostic tests (based on ICD-9-CM groupings) for patients discharged from short-stay hospitals (Table 7.9).

Table 7.9

Rates of High-Volume Procedures and Diagnostic Tests for Patients Discharged from Short-Stay Hospitals: United States, 1995

Procedure/Test	Rate per 100,000 Population
Computerized axial tomography	369.9
Diagnostic ultrasound	451.9
Cardiac catheterization	406.7
Cesarean section	300.2
Radioisotope scan	117.0
Arteriography and angiography using contrast material	701.5
Hysterectomy	222.9
Cholecystectomy	179.8
Colonoscopy and sigmoidoscopy	165.7
Endoscopy of small intestine	341.4
Endoscopy of large intestine	195.8
Prostatectomy	91.5
Coronary artery bypass graft	219.2
Excision or destruction of inter-vertebral disc and spinal fusion	104.5
Pacemaker insertion	120.0
Appendectomy	90.7

SOURCE: CDC/National Center for Health Statistics (1997c).

Ambulatory Care

In evaluating the provision of ambulatory care, one should consider studying conditions that are treated frequently in ambulatory settings. This is especially important for generating provider profiles, because such profiles are likely to be valid only if a single provider has a sufficient number of patients with the condition being profiled. Table 7.10 lists the most common reasons for outpatient visits in 1995.

Table 7.10

**Number and Percentage Distribution of Outpatient
Visits: United States, 1995**

Principal Diagnosis	Thousands of Visits	Percentage Distribution
All visits	67,232	100.0
General medical examination	3,831	5.7
Normal pregnancy	3,234	4.8
Cough	1,545	2.3
Postoperative visit	1,497	2.2
Throat symptoms	1,148	1.7
Stomach and abdominal pain	1,108	1.7
Well-baby examination	1,051	1.6
Earache or ear infection	984	1.5
Disorders of back	837	1.2
Essential hypertension	738	1.1
Diabetes mellitus	719	1.1

SOURCE: CDC/National Center for Health Statistics (1997b).

WHAT TARGET CONDITIONS SHOULD BE INCLUDED?

We have identified several conditions and procedures that clinical information system developers may wish to target for surveillance using the clinical data base. These conditions meet at least one of the specifications discussed above:

- Contributes significantly to morbidity and mortality of the population;

- Appropriate medical care for the condition has the potential to improve outcomes;

- A large proportion of the population is affected or involves high-volume procedures;

- Care is expensive, either because of medical charges or in lost work days; and

- Quality varies widely or is substandard.

Although not intended to be an exhaustive list, the target conditions listed below span the range of preventive/screening services, chronic conditions, and high-volume procedures.

Preventive/screening services

Breast cancer screening
Childhood immunizations
Adult immunizations
Prenatal/maternal care
Cervical cancer screening
Colorectal cancer screening
Smoking prevention
Hypertension screening
Cholesterol screening

Treatment of chronic conditions

Coronary artery disease
Hypertension
Stroke and cerebrovascular disease
Diabetes mellitus
Hip fracture
Otitis media
Childhood asthma
Depression

Procedures

Hysterectomy
Prostatectomy
Intervertebral disc excision and spinal fusion
Abdominal aortic aneurysm surgery
Cataract surgery

In the sections that follow, we specify the goals of surveillance and the reasons why surveillance is important for each target condition. When appropriate, we have noted where severity adjustment may be necessary. For two conditions, screening for breast cancer and treatment of cardiovascular disease, we have included specific additional questions analysts may wish to address, as well as data elements needed to answer those questions and current sources of the data. For these examples, the majority of data elements would come from a clinical information system. The detailed examples for breast cancer screening and treatment of cardiovascular disease are listed first, followed by the other target conditions. The purpose is to illustrate a process that can guide system design and planning.

DETAILED EXAMPLES FOR TWO TARGET CONDITIONS

Breast Cancer Screening

Overall Goal. Decrease the morbidity and mortality of breast cancer through early detection.

Objectives.

- Evaluate the rate of mammography screening among women over age 50;

- Evaluate the rate of clinical breast exam screening among women over age 50;

- Evaluate the rate of breast self-exams among women over age 50; and

- Evaluate the proportion of Stage I and II breast cancer diagnoses among total breast cancer diagnoses.

Rationale for Selecting Clinical Area. Breast cancer is a leading cause of death in women in the United States, with nearly 40,000 annual deaths (NCHS, 1990). Although primary prevention is at this time not possible, you can reduce the morbidity and mortality of breast cancer through early detection using mammography, clinical breast examination, and breast self-examination. The National Cancer Institute (NCI) has set the goal for the nation that, by the year 2000, 80 percent of women ages 50 to 70 would receive annual breast exams (NCI Breast Cancer Screening Consortium, 1990). Nationally, about 35 percent of women over age 40 report having had a mammogram within the past year. Forty-nine percent report having had one in the past three years. A much lower percentage of women over age 50, 26 percent, report having had a mammogram within the past three years (Anderson and May, 1995). Lower-than-ideal rates of screening mammography, clinical breast examination, and breast self-examination may result from inadequate access to services, lack of knowledge about the benefits of the screening, or failure of the health care system to encourage screening. If lower-than-optimal rates of screening are found, these are potential areas of intervention to increase the overall rate of mammography screening.

Target Population. Women between the ages of 50 and 75.

Examples of Specific Questions.

Quality of care.

1. What is the rate of mammography screening for women over age 50 in a health plan or community, in the last year?

2. What is rate of annual clinical breast exams for women over age 50 in a health plan or community?

3. What percentage of breast cancer diagnoses among women older than age 50 are Stage I or II?

Access.

4. Is the rate of mammography screening equivalent for different racial/ethnic groups and for women of different SES or insurance type?

5. Is the rate of breast exams equivalent for different racial/ethnic groups and for women of different SES?

6. Does the percentage of Stage I or II breast cancer diagnoses vary with different racial/ethnic groups or for women of different SES or insurance type?

Cost and cost-effectiveness.

7. Is mammography screening cost-effective (i.e., what is the cost per additional year of life saved if the rate of screening is increased from 70 percent to 90 percent)? How does this compare with the costs of treating women with Stage III or higher cancer?

Performance of health plan and providers.

8. What is the rate of mammography screening for women over age 50 continuously enrolled in a health plan over the previous 12 months?

9. Does the rate differ for women from different racial/ethnic groups or SES?

10. What percentage of a provider's panel of continuously enrolled female patients over age 50 have received mammography screening in the past year (this assumes a panel of at least 100 women in the age range)?

11. What is the rate of annual clinical breast exams for women over age 50 continuously enrolled in the health plan over the previous 12 months?

12. What percentage of breast cancer diagnoses among women older than age 50 who have been enrolled at least 18 months are Stage I or II?

13. Does the percentage differ for women from different racial/ethnic groups or SES?

Effect of public health programs (if applicable).

14. How has a mobile mammography unit influenced the rate of mammography in a specific community?

Effect of policy changes (if applicable).

15. How has the addition of a copayment for mammograms influenced the rate of mammography screening in the health plan?

16. Does the effect differ for women from different racial/ethnic groups or SES?

Tables 7.11 and 7.12 illustrate an organizational framework for defining the necessary data elements for developing a clinical data set for breast cancer detection.

Treatment of Coronary Artery Disease

Overall Goal. Decrease morbidity and mortality among those with a diagnosis of coronary artery disease (CAD).

Objectives.

• Evaluate quality of care for patients with myocardial infarction;

• Evaluate quality of ambulatory care for persons with coronary artery disease;

• Evaluate appropriateness of angiography, percutaneous transluminal coronary angioplasty (PTCA), CABG surgery;

• Evaluate mortality from CABG surgery; and

• Evaluate quality of life in patients with coronary artery disease.

Rationale for Selecting Clinical Area. Despite recent reductions in mortality, coronary artery disease remains the leading cause of mortality in the United States (U.S. Public Health Service, 1990; Siu et al., 1992; CDC, 1997a), resulting in over 500,000 deaths per year at a cost of over $40 billion per year. Primary and secondary prevention of coronary artery disease rests, in part, in controlling hypertension, high blood cholesterol, and smoking. Tertiary prevention of morbidity and mortality in patients with established heart disease involves lowering cholesterol levels (Blankenhorn et al., 1987); treating chronic angina with beta-blockers (Yusuf et al., 1985); treating unstable angina with anti-coagulation (Theroux et al., 1988); appropriately using medical interventions, such as thrombolysis and angioplasty, in the acute treatment of myocardial infarction (Michels and Yusuf, 1995; Van de Werf, 1994); and effectively treating the post-acute presentation of myocardial infarction (Oldridge et al., 1988).

Table 7.11

Necessary Data Elements to Answer Questions Regarding Breast Cancer Detection Programs

Data Element	Generic/ Specific	Current Source	Purpose	Questions
Unique identifier	G	Enrollment	Track patients across systems	1–16
Gender	G	Enrollment	Identify all women in system	1–16
Age	G	Enrollment	Identify all women over age 50	1–16
Race/ethnicity	G	Enrollment	Identify women of specific race	4–6, 9, 13, 16
Education level	G	Enrollment	Identify women of differing SES for access and risk adjustment	4–6, 8–13, 16
Income	G	Enrollment	Identify women of differing SES for access and risk adjustment	4–6, 8–13, 16
Insurance	G	Enrollment and community survey	Identify insurance status	4–6
Date of enrollment	G	Enrollment	Identify enrollment status	1–16
Date of disenrollment	G	Enrollment	Identify enrollment status	1–16
Performance of screening mammogram	S	Encounter	Identify screening mammograms performed	1, 4, 7, 8–10, 13–16
Cost of screening mammogram	S	Other files	Calculate costs of screening program	7
Stage I breast cancer diagnosis	S	Medical record, pathology, cancer registry	Identify women with early breast cancer	3, 6, 12, 13
Stage II breast cancer diagnosis	S	Medical record, pathology, cancer registry	Identify women with early breast cancer	3, 6, 12, 13
Mortality from breast cancer within 5 years of diagnosis	S	Medical record, death certificate	Identify women who have died from breast cancer	7

Table 7.12

Examples of Derived Variables Needed to Answer Questions Regarding Breast Cancer Detection Programs

Derived Variable	Generic/ Specific	Current Source	Purpose	Questions
Number of women over age 50 continuously enrolled over past 12 months	S	Enrollment	Denominator for rate calculations	1, 8, 14, 15
Number of women over age 50 continuously enrolled over past 12 months with at least one mammogram in previous 12 months	S	Encounter plus enrollment	Specific numerator to use to calculate rates	1, 8, 14, 15
Number of black women over age 50 continuously enrolled over past 12 months	S	Enrollment	Denominator for rate calculations specific to race	4, 9, 16
Number of black women over age 50 continuously enrolled over past 12 months with at least one mammogram in previous 12 months	S	Encounter plus enrollment	Numerator for rate calculations specific to race	4, 9, 16
Sample of women over age 50 continuously enrolled over past 12 months	S	Enrollment (to identify sample)	Denominator for rate calculations	2, 11
Number of women in sample over age 50 continuously enrolled in plan over past 12 months with clinical breast exam in past 12 months	S	Enrollment (to identify sample) plus medical record (or survey)	Numerator for rate calculation	2, 11
Number of total breast cancer diagnoses in past year among women over age 50 enrolled in plan for at least 18 months before diagnosis	S	Enrollment plus medical record or cancer registry (if registry, use unique identifiers)	Denominator	3, 12
Number of Stage I and Stage II breast cancer diagnoses in past year among women over age 50 enrolled in plan for at least 18 months prior to their diagnosis	S	Enrollment plus medical record or cancer registry	Numerator to calculate proportion of breast cancer diagnoses that are Stage I and Stage II	3, 12

For example, Siu et al. (1992) demonstrated that increasing use of thrombolytic treatment from 40 to 75 percent of eligible patients would reduce mortality by 9.3 percent and reduce the annual number of deaths by 1,172. Similarly, use of beta-blockers after myocardial infarction reduces the risk of death by an estimated 22 percent (Yusuf et al., 1988). Increasing the percentage of eligible postinfarction patients treated with beta-blockers from 40 percent to 75 percent could reduce the annual number of deaths nationally by over 1,800 (Siu et al., 1992). Although increasing use of appropriate treatment may reduce morbidity and mortality, several studies have demonstrated that some procedures (e.g., PTCA and CABG surgery) may be performed for inappropriate medical indications (Hilborne et al., 1993; Leape et al., 1993). Finally, recent studies have demonstrated lower rates of interventions for coronary disease among blacks, suggesting differences in access to treatment (Wenneker and Epstein, 1989; Carlisle et al., 1995; Carlisle et al., 1997; Peterson et al., 1997).

Target Population. Men and women with known or suspected coronary artery disease.

Examples of Specific Questions.

Quality of care.

Process

1. What percentage of patients with indications for thrombolytic therapy at time of admission received thrombolysis within two hours of admission?

2. What percentage of eligible patients with myocardial infarction were discharged on beta-blocker therapy?

3. What percentage of patients with myocardial infarction had a follow-up visit within one month of discharge?

4. What percentage of hypertensive patients with known CAD had well controlled hypertension (all values less than 140/90) in the preceding year?

5. What percentage of smokers with known coronary disease were counseled regarding smoking cessation at least once within the preceding year?

Outcomes

6. What is the severity-adjusted 30-day mortality rate for patients admitted with myocardial infarction?

7. What is the severity-adjusted 30-day mortality rate after CABG surgery?

8. What is the severity-adjusted quality of life for patients with known coronary artery disease?

9. What is the severity-adjusted quality of life and functional status for patients after CABG surgery?

Appropriateness

10. What percentage of cardiac procedures (angiography, PTCA, CABG) were performed for appropriate indications?

11. Did everyone who could benefit from a procedure get one?

Access.

12. Is there a difference in adequacy of blood pressure control for CAD patients of lower versus higher SES (severity-stratified)?

13. Is there differential underuse of cardiac procedures (angiography, PTCA, or CABG) across SES groups?

Costs and cost-effectiveness.

14. What are the severity-adjusted costs of CABG surgery in one hospital versus another?

15. What is the severity-adjusted cost-effectiveness of rehabilitation programs after myocardial infarction?

Performance of health plan and providers.

16. What percentage of the health plan's hypertensive patients with known CAD had well-controlled hypertension (all values less than 140/90) in the preceding year?

17. What percentage of the health plan's smokers with known coronary disease were counseled regarding smoking cessation at least once within the preceding year?

18. What is the severity-adjusted 30-day mortality rate after CABG for all patients in the health plan?

19. What is the severity-adjusted 30-day mortality rate after CABG by individual surgeons?

Effect of public health programs on health (if applicable).

20. Does imposition of a cigarette tax decrease the proportion of smokers among persons with known CAD?

Effect of policy changes on health (if applicable).

21. How did a newly instituted preauthorization program change the utilization profile for angioplasty (severity-adjusted)?

Table 7.13 illustrates an organizational framework for defining the necessary
data elements for developing a clinical data set for treatment of cardiovascular
disease.

ADDITIONAL TARGET CONDITIONS FOR CONSIDERATION

The following target conditions are divided into

- Preventive/screening services;

- Treatment of chronic conditions; and

- Procedures.

Goals of evaluation and reasons why the condition should be considered for
evaluation are provided. Evaluations could focus on the specific areas previously defined (quality of care, access to care, cost and cost-effectiveness, performance of health plan and providers, effect of public health programs on
health, and effect of policy changes on health).

When possible, evaluations should include all population groups and may also
be divided by gender, race/ethnicity, or socioeconomic status to assess possible
differences in access to care. Results of new studies and publication of new
recommendations need to be reviewed regularly in an effort to update indicators.

This list is meant to serve as a guide for choosing indicators and is not intended
to be exhaustive. Areas not included on this list may also be appropriate for
evaluation. Similarly, clinical information system developers need not choose
all of the target areas listed below.

Preventive/Screening Services

Childhood Immunizations.

Overall goal.

Reduce morbidity and mortality from preventable infectious diseases among
children through appropriate immunization.

Table 7.13

Necessary Data Elements to Answer Questions Regarding Treatment of Cardiovascular Disease

Data Element	Generic/ Specific	Current Source	Purpose	Questions
Unique identifier	G	Enrollment	Track patients across systems	1–21
Gender	G	Enrollment	Risk adjustment/access to care evaluation	6–9, 12–15, 18–21
Age	G	Enrollment	Risk adjustment	6–9, 12–15, 18–21
Race/ethnicity	G	Enrollment	Access to care evaluation/ risk adjustment	11–13
Education level	G	Enrollment	Identify patients of differing SES for access and risk adjustment	11–13
Income	G	Enrollment	Identify patients of differing SES for access and risk adjustment	11–13
Insurance	G	Enrollment and community survey	Identify insurance status	11–13
Date of enrollment	G	Enrollment	Identify enrollment status	16–19
Date of disenrollment	G	Enrollment	Identify enrollment status	16–19
Provider unique identifier	G	Encounter	Evaluation of providers	19
Facility unique identifier	G	Encounter	Evaluation of facilities	16–18
Coronary artery disease diagnosis indicated by the presence of one or more of the following: — coded diagnosis of coronary artery disease, myocardial infarction, angina pectoris, ischemic cardiomyopathy — positive exercise stress test — angiogram with at least 70% narrowing in one or more vessels	S	Encounter/medical record	Identify patients with coronary artery disease	1–21

Table 7.13 (continued)

Data Element	Generic/Specific	Current Source	Purpose	Questions
Presence of hypertension	S	Medical record	Identify patients with hypertension for process of care evaluations and risk adjustment	4,12,16
Control of hypertension (all blood pressure readings in last year <140/90) (derived)	S	Medical record	Process of care evaluation	4,12,16
Smoking history	S	Medical record	Identify past and present smokers; risk adjustment	5,17
Current smoking	S	Medical record	Process of care evaluation	5,17
Counseled regarding smoking in last year	S	Medical record/survey	Process of care evaluation	5,17
Time of previous myocardial infarction	S	Medical record	Risk adjustment	7,9,10
Diabetes	G	Medical record/encounter	Risk adjustment	7,10,11,13,18,19
Dialysis dependence	S	Medical record/encounter	Risk adjustment	7,10,11,13,18,19
Indications for surgery	S	Angiography report/medical record	Appropriateness evaluation/risk adjustment	7,10,11,13,18,19
— left main disease				
— number of diseased vessels				
— proximal left anterior descending artery stenosis				
Class of angina	S	Medical record/survey	Appropriateness evaluation/risk adjustment	7,10,11,13,18,19
Exercise stress test results	S	Cardiodiagnostic report/medical record	Appropriateness evaluation	7,10,11,13,18,19
Number of previous CABG surgeries	S	Medical record	Risk adjustment	7,10,11,13,18,19
Left ventricular ejection fraction (percent)	S	Echocardiogram/angiography reports	Risk adjustment	7,10,11,13,18,19

Table 7.13 (continued)

Data Element	Generic/Specific	Current Source	Purpose	Questions
Unstable angina	S	Medical record	Risk adjustment	7,10,11,13,18,19
Congestive heart failure	S	Medical record/encounter	Risk adjustment	7,10,11,13,18,19
Valve operation	S	Medical record/encounter	Risk adjustment	7,10,11,13,18,19
Preoperative intra-aortic balloon pump	S	Medical record	Risk adjustment	7,10,11,13,18,19
30-day postsurgical mortality	S	Medical record/death certificate	Outcome evaluation	7,18,19
30-day postmyocardial infarction mortality	S	Medical record/death certificate	Outcome evaluation	6
Comorbid conditions	G	Medical record/encounter	Risk adjustment	
Pre-admission functional status	S	Survey	Outcome evaluation	8,9
Pre-admission quality of life	S	Survey	Outcome evaluation	8,9
Postsurgical or postdischarge functional status	S	Survey	Outcome evaluation	8,9
Postsurgical or postdischarge quality of life	S	Survey	Outcome evaluation	8,9
Diagnosis of acute myocardial infarction on admission	S	Medical record/encounter	Identify patients with acute myocardial infarction	1,2,3,6
Eligibility for thrombolysis (e.g., EKG changes, pain lasting less than 6 hours, no contraindications)	S	Medical record	Identify patients eligible for procedure	1
Thrombolysis	S	Medical record	Process of care evaluation	1
Treatment with beta-blocker medication post myocardial infarction (derived)	S	Medical record/pharmacy file	Process of care evaluation	2
Follow-up within 2 weeks after discharge for myocardial infarction (derived)	S	Medical record/encounter	Process of care evaluation	3

Objectives.

- Evaluate rates of immunization for MMR, OPV, DPT, influenza type B, varicella (chicken pox), and hepatitis B among children under age two for all population groups.

- Evaluate morbidity and mortality caused by preventable infections.

Rationale for selecting clinical area.

Ten infectious diseases are preventable by childhood vaccination: diphtheria, pertussis, and tetanus; measles, mumps, and rubella; polio; *Haemophilus influenzae* type B; hepatitis B ; and varicella (U.S. Public Health Service, 1994).

In fact, 80 percent of all immunizations recommended for children should be administered during the child's first two years of life (CDC, 1994a). Yet, national estimates from 1992 indicated that only 82.5 percent of children age two were vaccinated against measles; 83 percent against diphtheria, pertussis, and tetanus; and 72.4 percent against polio. Children who were either poor or black had lower rates of vaccination (CDC, 1994a). Overall, in 1992, only 71.6 percent of two-year-olds had received their full set of vaccinations (Robinson et al., 1994). The National Committee for Quality Assurance reports that, on average, the health plans that collect Health Plan Employer Data and Information Set (HEDIS) data currently have average rates for a more comprehensive vaccine series (four DPT, three OPV, one MMR, one influenza type B, and two hepatitis B) of 59 to 81 percent (NCQA, 1997a).

Inadequate childhood vaccination received attention when a marked increase in the incidence of measles was attributed to a failure to vaccinate children by their second birthday (U.S. Public Health Service, 1994). In response, the U.S. Public Health Service recommended that the basic immunization series be administered to at least 90 percent of all children under age two, and to 95 percent of children in licensed child care facilities, kindergarten, or postsecondary education institutions (U.S. Public Health Service, 1990). As of 1995, the U.S. Preventive Services Task Force (USPSTF) recommended that all children without established contraindications receive DPT, OPV, MMR, influenza type B, hepatitis B, and varicella vaccinations at scheduled intervals beginning at age two months and ending at age six years. They also recommended that a tetanus-diphtheria (Td) booster be administered at age 14–16, and then periodically throughout adulthood (USPSTF, 1995).

Adult Immunizations.

Overall goal.

Reduce morbidity and mortality from preventable infectious disease among adults through appropriate immunization.

Objectives.

- Evaluate rates of immunization for pneumonia and influenza among people age 65 and older.

- Evaluate rates of immunization for pneumonia and influenza among those at increased risk of serious consequences from these diseases.

- Evaluate mortality and hospitalization rates from epidemic-related pneumonia and influenza among people age 65 and older (severity-adjusted).

Rationale for selecting clinical area.

The USPSTF recommends that (1) pneumococcal vaccine (pneumovax) be administered at least once to all immunocompetent individuals who are age 65 or older or who are at high risk and may be readministered after six or more years or if the previous immunization occurred before 1983 (i.e., the person received an older version of the vaccine); and (2) influenza vaccine be administered annually (at the start of the flu season) to those who are age 65 or older or who are in specific high-risk groups (USPSTF, 1995).

Acute respiratory conditions such as pneumonia and influenza were the sixth leading cause of death in the United States and accounted for over 80,000 deaths in 1993. The majority of these deaths (89 percent) were among people age 65 or older (NCHS, 1994). Additionally, an estimated 2,000 to 8,000 deaths can occur in this age group during an influenza epidemic (Lui et al., 1987). Influenza can be prevented by annual vaccination before the start of flu season, and vaccination can be especially helpful in preventing hospitalization, pneumonia, and death among higher-risk individuals such as older adults and those with certain chronic conditions (Arden et al., 1993). In fact, influenza immunization could reduce mortality in the elderly population as much as 59 percent (Gross et al., 1988). Each year, however, less than 30 percent of individuals in high-risk groups are immunized against influenza (Arden et al., 1993). Influenza immunization among the elderly has increased in recent years, with as many as 58 percent of adults over age 65 reporting influenza immunization in 1995 (CDC, 1997b). As stated above, it is recommended that the pneumococcal vaccine be given only as a one-time dose. Like influenza, vaccination against pneumonia is an effective way to prevent disease especially for older people, yet, in 1995, only 35.6 percent of adults age 65 and over had ever received the pneumococcal vaccine (CDC, 1997b). The U.S. Public Health Service identified this problem of underimmunization and set forth a national objective for the year 2000 of vaccinating at least 60 percent of noninstitutionalized high-risk individuals (and 80 percent of institutionalized chronically ill or older people) against pneumonia and influenza (U.S. Public Health Service, 1990).

Prenatal/Maternal Care.

Overall goals.

- Reduce neonatal morbidity and mortality through prenatal care and counseling.

- Reduce maternal morbidity and mortality through prenatal care and appropriate use of procedures.

Objectives.

- Evaluate the percentage of pregnancies with appropriate prenatal care for all population groups.

- Evaluate the percentage of infants with low birthweights (severity-adjusted) for all population groups.

- Determine rates of cesarean section deliveries and appropriateness of cesarean section.

Rationale for selecting clinical area.

Although infant mortality occurs in fewer than 11 per 1,000 live births, low birthweights (less than 2,500 grams), which predict both short-term and long-term infant morbidity, account for 6 percent of all live births. Adequate prenatal care improves pregnancy outcomes, especially for women at increased medical or social risk (U.S. Public Health Service, 1990). Prenatal care includes screening for anemia and sexually transmitted diseases, determination of fetal age and size, appropriate genetic screening and counseling, and management of pregnancy-related complications. Murata et al. (1994) have reviewed the literature on this topic and made specific recommendations regarding process criteria that should be included in evaluating the quality of prenatal care. Such criteria may be used to determine (1) the adequacy of care provided by individual health care providers or health systems, (2) access to prenatal care for different population subgroups, and (3) the effect of policy changes (such as reimbursement rates) on quality of prenatal care.

Cesarean sections accounted for approximately 23 percent of all deliveries in 1993, a rate that is the lowest in the United States since 1985, but one that is still almost four times the rate in 1970 (CDC, 1995). Recent data indicate that many cesarean sections may be unnecessary (Flamm et al., 1988; Stewart et al., 1990) and contribute to maternal morbidity and mortality (Lilford et al., 1990; Miller, 1988). Appropriate indications for cesarean sections have been developed (ACOG, 1994) and an evaluation of cesarean section rates and appropriateness of cesarean sections may lead to policy changes advocating more appropriate cesarean section use.

Cervical Cancer Screening.

Overall goal.

Reduce morbidity and mortality through early detection and appropriate treatment.

Objectives.

- Evaluate the rate of screening Pap smears in women ages 18 to 64 in past two years for all population groups.

- Evaluate the appropriateness of follow-up for abnormal Pap smears for all population groups.

- Evaluate the incidence of invasive cervical cancer.

- Determine the cervical cancer mortality rate in women ages 18 to 64 per 100,000 women in the same age group.

Rationale for selecting clinical area.

Cervical cancer incidence and mortality decreased more than 70 percent from 1950 to 1987. This rapid decline was attributed to the introduction of the Pap smear, which enables the disease to be detected in an extremely early and highly treatable stage (NCI, 1988). Even so, the U.S. Public Health Service has established a national objective for the year 2000 to further decrease cervical cancer mortality rates by more than 50 percent (U.S. Public Health Service, 1990). The U.S. Preventive Services Task Force recommends

- That all women who are or who ever have been sexually active receive regular Pap tests, or by the time they turn 18;

- That these tests begin when a woman becomes sexually active and be performed at least every three years, at the physician's discretion, depending on the presence of certain risk factors; and

- That Pap smears be discontinued when the woman reaches age 65 if previous tests have consistently been normal (USPSTF, 1995).

The U.S. Public Health Service stated that by the year 2000 the proportion of women age 18 or older who have ever obtained a Pap smear should increase to 95 percent (from a 1987 baseline of 88 percent), and the proportion of women who received a Pap test some time within the previous three years should increase to 85 percent (from a 1987 baseline of 75 percent). In fact, specific groups such as Hispanic women, women with less than a high school education, women with low incomes, and women age 70 or older were identified as special target populations because their current rates of Pap testing were below average (U.S. Public Health Service, 1990).

Colorectal Cancer Screening.

Overall goal.

Reduce morbidity and mortality from colorectal cancer.

Objectives.

- Evaluate the rate of colorectal cancer screening by sigmoidoscopy or fecal occult blood testing (FOBT) for adults age 50 and older for all population groups.

- Evaluate the incidence of advanced stage colorectal cancer for all population groups.

Rationale for selecting clinical area.

In 1990, approximately 155,000 new cases of colorectal cancer were diagnosed, and slightly more than 60,000 people were estimated to have died from colorectal cancer. These numbers represent about 15 percent of all cancers diagnosed and 12 percent of all deaths from cancer. The trend since 1950 shows an increase of approximately 19 percent in the incidence and a decrease of approximately 20 percent in the mortality, which is probably due to earlier diagnosis and treatment (NCI, 1988). Even so, colorectal cancer is the second most common cancer and has the second highest mortality rate in the United States (USPSTF, 1995). Primary prevention of colorectal cancer, or prevention of the cancer before it ever happens, has been examined with respect to diet modifications, but thus far the results have been inconclusive. Therefore, the greatest effect on reducing mortality and morbidity from colorectal cancer is through secondary prevention (Siu et al., 1992).

There are three possible screening tests for early detection of colorectal cancer—digital rectal examination, FOBT, and rigid or flexible sigmoidoscopy. The
efficacy of these tests to detect cancer in asymptomatic individuals is somewhat
controversial. The digital rectal exam is of limited value because it detects less
than 10 percent of colorectal cancers. The sensitivity of FOBT is reported to
be anywhere from 26 to 92 percent, and its specifity about 90 to 99 percent. The
high false positive rate of FOBT results in potentially unnecessary and
expensive follow-up tests. Forthcoming studies of FOBT include new assays,
which may improve its sensitivity, and the use of FOBT in combination with
sigmoidoscopy as a screening tool. Sigmoidoscopy, which is the most
expensive and least pleasant of the screening tests, can detect anywhere from
25 to 30 percent (rigid sigmoidoscope) to 40 to 65 percent (60–65 cm long
flexible sigmoidoscope) of colorectal cancers. Whether increasing the length to
105 cm also increases the detection rate is currently being evaluated. However,
sigmoidoscopy may also yield false positive results because it can detect polyps
that may never become malignant (USPSTF, 1995). Yet, several studies have
demonstrated definite benefits in mortality from periodic screening by
sigmoidoscopy (Friedman and Selby, 1990; Selby et al., 1992). Thus, the recommendations for screening also remain somewhat controversial.

The American Cancer Society recommends annual digital rectal exams for all
adults age 40 or older, annual FOBT beginning at age 50, and sigmoidoscopy
every 3–5 years beginning at age 50. The USPSTF recommends annual colorectal cancer screening for persons age 50 or over but does not specify which of the
two preferred methods, FOBT or sigmoidoscopy, should be used (USPSTF,
1995). Although the issue of how best to screen for this disease remains controversial, it will continue to receive attention because the U.S. Public Health
Service has targeted colorectal cancer deaths to be reduced to no more than
13.2 per 100,000 people by the year 2000 (U.S. Public Health Service, 1990).

Smoking Prevention.

Overall goal.

To reduce morbidity and mortality from lung disease, heart disease, and stroke
by reducing smoking prevalence.

Objectives.

- Evaluate cigarette smoking prevalence in the community/health plan by
  age, race, and gender.

- Evaluate the use of educational programs, physician counseling, and public
  health programs to reduce smoking prevalence.

- Evaluate the efficacy of educational programs over time.

Rationale for selecting clinical area.

Although cigarette smoking has decreased over the past 25 years, one-quarter of adults in the United States smoke and more than three-quarters of smokers begin when they are teenagers. In addition, cigarette smoking is more common among men, American Indians, Eskimos, and Aleuts, and individuals of lower socioeconomic status. It has become almost as prevalent among women as men (USPSTF, 1995). Smoking is the attributable cause of approximately one in five deaths in the United States, and it affects many areas of morbidity and mortality, including cancers of the respiratory system and some internal organs, heart and cerebrovascular diseases, lung disease for both the smoker and the passive or involuntary smoker, and morbidity for infants of mothers who smoke. In addition, smoking is responsible for fire-related deaths and injuries (USPSTF, 1995).

Smoking cessation programs have been shown to improve by 5.8 percent a smoker's chances of remaining off cigarettes after 12 months (Kottke et al., 1988). Although smoking is considered to be the most modifiable cause of death, and clinicians have both the opportunity and the means to modify smoking behavior in their patients, several studies have shown that many physicians fail to advise their patients to quit. For this reason, one recommendation of the USPSTF is that tobacco counseling be offered regularly to all patients who smoke (cigarettes, pipes, or cigars) and to those who use smokeless tobacco. The prescription of nicotine patches or gums is recommended as an adjunct to counseling. In addition, the USPSTF recommends that adolescents and young adults who do not currently use tobacco products be targeted and advised not to start (USPSTF, 1995).

Hypertension Screening.

Overall goal.

To reduce morbidity and mortality from coronary artery disease, stroke, and kidney disease through early identification of hypertension.

Objective.

* Evaluate the percentage of adults (age 18 and older) with at least one blood pressure measurement in previous years, separately by population group.

Rationale for selecting clinical area.

Siu et al. (1992) estimated that at least 18 percent of the adult population have definite hypertension (systolic $\geq$ 160 mm Hg and diastolic $\geq$ 95 mm Hg) and approximately 30 percent have blood pressure readings of greater than 140/90 mm Hg (NHLBI, 1985; U.S. Public Health Service, 1990). Hypertension or high blood pressure is a leading risk factor for coronary artery disease, congestive heart failure, stroke, and cerebrovascular disease (USPSTF, 1995). Long-term blood pressure control has been shown to help reduce the incidence of and death caused by cerebrovascular diseases (U.S. Public Health Service, 1990). For instance, one study found that the incidence of stroke could be reduced by an estimated 40 percent through treatment of mild-to-moderate hypertension (Herbert et al., 1988). Similarly, if the average diastolic blood pressure for persons with hypertension was reduced by 5 to 6 mm Hg, the incidence of coronary artery disease could be reduced by 14 percent and the incidence of strokes could be reduced by 42 percent (USPSTF, 1995). In parallel with this information, the U.S. Public Health Service's objectives for the year 2000 are that at least 50 percent of people with high blood pressure have their blood pressure under control (less than 140 mm Hg systolic and 90 mm Hg diastolic) and at least 90 percent of people with high blood pressure are taking action to get their pressure under control (U.S. Public Health Service, 1990).

To better identify and treat hypertension, the USPSTF recommends that

- Blood pressure be measured regularly to screen for hypertension in all individuals who are age three or older;

- In adults over 21 years of age, the measurements be made at least once every two years if the last blood pressure readings were less than 140 mm Hg systolic and 85 mm Hg diastolic, and annually if the last diastolic blood pressure was 85 to 89 mm Hg;

- Hypertension be diagnosed after more than one reading exceeding either threshold at each of three separate visits; and

- Once hypertension is confirmed, the patient receive counseling about exercise, weight reduction, dietary sodium intake, and alcohol consumption (USPSTF, 1995).

Cholesterol Screening.

Overall goal.

To reduce morbidity and mortality from coronary artery disease through detection of hypercholesterolemia.

Objective.

- Evaluate the percentage of adults with at least one cholesterol measurement in previous five years, separately by population group.

Rationale for selecting clinical area.

Coronary artery disease is the leading cause of death in the United States and high blood cholesterol, along with cigarette smoking and hypertension, are the principal modifiable risk factors (USPSTF, 1995). In fact, the progression of established coronary artery disease can be slowed by lowering plasma cholesterol (Blankenhorn et al., 1987). Therefore, blood cholesterol measurement identifies those who need treatment for high cholesterol and it provides an opportunity for counseling about ways to reduce risk of coronary artery disease (U.S. Public Health Service, 1990). The U.S. Public Health Service stated that, by the year 2000, at least three-quarters of all adults should have had their blood cholesterol checked within the preceding five years (U.S. Public Health Service, 1990). In addition, the USPSTF recommends that

- Periodic measurements of total serum cholesterol be made for all men ages 35 to 65, and for women ages 45 to 65; periodic screening may also be considered for certain persons over age 65, such as those with other CAD risk factors;

- The interval of these measurements be left to clinical discretion although every five years was suggested for all except those with prior evidence of elevated cholesterol; and

- All patients periodically receive counseling about dietary intake of fat (especially saturated fat) and cholesterol (USPSTF, 1995).

Although there is considerable evidence that high blood cholesterol levels are associated with an increased risk of coronary artery disease among young and middle-aged adults, the evidence for the association among older adults is somewhat controversial. A recent study reported that, among older adults (over age 70), elevated blood cholesterol levels were not associated with a significantly higher rate of mortality from coronary artery disease (Krumholtz et al., 1994).

Treatment of Chronic Conditions

Hypertension.

Overall goal.

Decrease morbidity and mortality from coronary artery disease, stroke, and kidney disease through control of hypertension.

Objective.

- Evaluate the percentage of patients with hypertension whose blood pressure is under control (≤ 140/90 mm Hg)

Rationale for selecting clinical area.

Hypertension is a major modifiable risk factor for coronary artery disease, stroke, and kidney disease. In fact, people with high blood pressure have three to four times the risk of developing coronary artery disease and up to seven times the risk of stroke as those persons who have normal blood pressure (Dawber, 1980; U.S. Public Health Service, 1990). Yet fewer than 50 percent of patients with hypertension have achieved good blood pressure control (U.S. Public Health Service, 1990). Control of blood pressure may be achieved through life-style modification (reduced salt intake, weight loss, and exercise) as well as medications. The U.S. Public Health Service has set as a goal for the year 2000 that 50 percent of all persons with hypertension (> 140/90 mm Hg) have their blood pressure under control (U.S. Public Health Service, 1990).

Stroke and Cerebrovascular Disease.

Overall goal.

Decrease morbidity and mortality from cerebrovascular disease.

Objectives.

- Evaluate blood pressure control.
- Evaluate the appropriateness of carotid endarterectomy for all population groups.
- Evaluate the use of aspirin for patients with transient ischemic attacks (TIAs) and previous strokes.

Rationale for selecting clinical area.

Heart disease and stroke kill nearly as many Americans as all other diseases combined (NCHS, 1994; U.S. Public Health Service, 1990) and are among the leading causes of disability. Cerebrovascular disease was the fourth leading cause of in-hospital death in 1992 (CDC, 1994b). Control of blood pressure, treatment of TIAs with aspirin (Barnett, 1994) and appropriate use of carotid endarterectomy (Haynes et al., 1994; Hobson et al., 1993) have been shown to have the greatest effect on reducing stroke incidence.

Diabetes Mellitus.

Overall goal.

Decrease morbidity and mortality from diabetes mellitus.

Objectives.

- Evaluate glycemic control.

- Evaluate the use of secondary preventive services in diabetes (retinal exams, podiatry care, hypertension control, and education).

- Evaluate mortality for diabetic complications (ketoacidosis, gangrene, and infections).

Rationale for selecting clinical area.

Diabetes is both prevalent and highly debilitating. Over 5.5 million Americans have been diagnosed with diabetes, and 300,000 die from the disease annually. Diabetes causes an estimated 5,800 cases of blindness, 40,000 amputations, and 4,000 cases of renal failure annually (Mazze et al. , 1985). Tight glycemic control of diabetes has been shown to reduce morbidity from diabetes (DCCT Research Group, 1993). Further, prevention of long-term complications may be possible apart from tight control. Careful annual retinal exams and appropriate treatment may reduce the incidence of blindness (Early Treatment Diabetic Retinopathy Study Research Group, 1985). Treatment of hypertension (Parving et al., 1983) and of microalbuminuria (Marre et al., 1988) may slow progression to renal failure. Patient education regarding foot care and smoking may be important in reducing the incidence of foot infection and cardiovascular disease (Browner, 1986). Similarly, control of hypertension and cholesterol reduction reduces the risk of cardiovascular disease.

Hip Fracture.

Overall goal.

Improve quality of life/functioning after hip fracture.

Objectives.

- Evaluate the quality of inpatient care (deep vein thrombosis prophylaxis, rates of infection, and rates of cardiac complications) given to persons with hip fractures for all population groups (severity-adjusted).

- Evaluate the quality of life after hip fracture, including functional status at three months.

Rationale for selecting clinical area.

Over 270,000 adults suffer hip fractures annually (CDC, 1994b). Fractures among older adults are associated with high mortality and often result in long-term care placement (Kelsey and Hoffman, 1987). Although prevention of hip fractures is difficult, appropriate treatment after fracture occurs may have an important effect on mortality and quality of life (Siu et al., 1992). Such treatment may include rehabilitation services, thrombophlebitis prophylaxis, and prevention and treatment of postsurgical complications.

Otitis Media with Effusion.

Overall goal.

Decrease hearing loss in patients with otitis media.

Objectives.

- Evaluate the appropriateness of antibiotic treatment and surgical procedures for children with otitis media with effusion.

- Evaluate the appropriateness of hearing evaluation in children with otitis media with effusion.

- Evaluate the incidence of hearing loss (> 20 dB bilaterally) among otitis-prone children.

Rationale for selecting clinical area.

Otitis media is the most common diagnosis for physician office visits by children under age 15 (Schappert, 1992). Approximately 30 percent of these visits are for otitis media with effusion (OME) (Stool et al., 1994), which is characterized by the presence of fluid in the middle ear without signs or symptoms of infection. If improperly treated, OME can result in hearing loss and delays in hearing-related development. The Agency for Health Care Policy and Research reviewed the literature and convened expert panels to develop guidelines for the optimal management of OME (Stool et al., 1994), including appropriate use of observation, antibiotics, and surgical intervention.

Childhood Asthma.

Overall goal.

Decrease morbidity and increase functional status in patients with asthma.

Objectives.

- Evaluate the process of ambulatory care (appropriateness of medication use, follow-up visits at regular intervals and after hospitalizations, and education) for children with asthma.

- Evaluate the rate of emergency department use.

- Evaluate the hospitalization rate for asthma exacerbations.

- Evaluate the functional status, disease-related patient knowledge, and quality of life for children with asthma.

Rationale for selecting clinical area.

Approximately 10.5 percent of children have at least one episode of asthma by the age of 17 (Friday and Fireman, 1988) and children with severe asthma miss more than twice as many school days as children without asthma (Parcel et al., 1979). Appropriate treatment and patient education have been shown to significantly reduce rates of asthma exacerbations, emergency room (ER) visits, hospitalizations, and lost school days (Siu et al., 1992). An example of such appropriate treatment is the use of short-term steroids in combination with other drugs early in the course of upper respiratory infection (Brunette et al., 1988). Further, rates of ER use may reflect poor access to primary care, and hospitalization rates may reflect poor access to or poor quality of ambulatory care. Most measurements should focus on process of care, but an evaluation of outcomes in the form of functional status and quality of life for children with asthma is also appropriate.

Depression.

Overall goal.

Decrease morbidity from major depression.

Objectives.

- Evaluate the detection of major depression in the primary care setting for all populations.

- Evaluate the appropriate use of medications and specialty referrals for depression for all populations.

Rationale for selecting clinical area.

The Agency for Health Care Policy and Research has published a clinical practice guideline on the detection, diagnosis, and treatment of depression in primary care (Depression Guideline Panel, 1993a, 1993b). The recommendations are based on extensive literature reviews and expert opinions. The panel found that approximately 3 percent of men and 6 percent of women in Western industrialized nations suffer from major depression at any point in time (Depression Guideline Panel, 1993a). The costs associated with depression (treatment and indirect costs from lost productivity) are significant—approximately $16 billion dollars per year in 1980 dollars. Despite its high prevalence, depression is both underdiagnosed and undertreated by primary care providers—less than one-half of persons with major depression are properly recognized. Yet, once identified, depression can most often be successfully treated (Depression Guideline Panel, 1993b). Therefore, to reach the goal of decreasing morbidity from depression, the focus should be on detection and appropriate treatment.

Procedures

The following procedures are highly prevalent, relatively expensive, and sometimes performed for inappropriate indications. In many cases, some patients who would benefit from these procedures may not receive them. An evaluation of rates and appropriateness may reveal issues related to quality of care, access, and performance that need to be addressed.

You could ask the following questions for any of the following operations:

- What percentage of surgeries were performed for appropriate indications?

- Did everyone who could benefit from the surgery get it?

- Did certain subgroups (i.e., high versus low SES or PPO versus HMO) of the population undergo surgery at higher or lower rates?

- What are the costs associated with surgery and is surgery cost-effective?

Hysterectomy. Over 500,000 hysterectomies are performed every year in the United States (Graves, 1991). The estimated cost of these hysterectomies is over $2 billion. There have been several reports, dating as far back as 1948, that a significant number of hysterectomies are performed for inappropriate indications (Doyle, 1953; DeFriese et al., 1989; Dyck et al., 1977; Jenkins, 1977; Miller, 1946). The American College of Obstetricians and Gynecologists (ACOG) has issued guidelines regarding the appropriate indications for hysterectomy (ACOG, 1989). Bernstein et al. (1993) found that an average of 16 percent of women across seven managed care plans underwent hysterectomy for inappropriate indications (range 10 to 27 percent).

Prostatectomy in Patients with Benign Prostatic Hypertrophy. The U.S. Department of Health and Human Services published guidelines on treatment of benign prostatic hypertrophy (BPH), which includes indications for surgery

(McConnell et al., 1994). The guidelines state that one in every four men in the United States will be treated for the relief of symptomatic BPH by age 80, and that over 300,000 surgical procedures for BPH, mostly transurethral resection (TURP), are performed annually. Although there are many treatment options for BPH, surgery offers the best chance for symptom improvement, but it also has the highest complication rate. The guidelines list specific indications for surgery.

Intervertebral Disc Excision and Spinal Fusion. Back problems are the most common reason for office visits to orthopedic surgeons, neurosurgeons, and occupational medicine physicians (Bigos et al., 1994). However, there is some evidence that many patients with low back pain may be receiving care that is inappropriate. A guideline published by AHCPR (Bigos et al., 1994) lists the indications for surgery in persons with low back pain and concludes that over 95 percent of persons presenting with acute low back pain will not benefit from surgery.

Abdominal Aortic Aneurysm Surgery. The Academic Medical Center Consortium, the American Medical Association, and RAND published a summary statement regarding the appropriate indications for abdominal aortic aneurysm surgery (Ballard et al., 1992). In an extensive literature review, they found that over 50,000 such surgeries are performed annually in the United States at a cost of over $1 billion. Since screening for an abdominal aortic aneurysm is relatively easy, the number of operations could potentially increase. Therefore, it may be useful to determine appropriateness of surgery.

Cataract Surgery. The Academic Medical Center Consortium, the American Medical Association, and RAND published a summary statement regarding the appropriate indications for cataract surgery (Lee et al., 1993). According to their literature review, cataract surgery is one of the most frequently performed surgical procedures in the United States and is the most frequently reimbursed procedure by Medicare. Between 1972 and 1977, the rate of cataract surgery increased by 39 percent, whereas the Medicare population increased by only 11 percent. Coincident with this increase was the development of new technologies, making cataract surgery more effective. A study in 10 academic medical centers found that 2 percent of cataract surgeries were inappropriate and 7 percent were of uncertain clinical value (Tobacman et al., 1996).

CAN A CLINICAL INFORMATION SYSTEM ANSWER ALL CLINICAL QUESTIONS?

A clinical information system allows you to capture essential data elements for defined clinical conditions to answer specific questions. An integrated data base would be a vast improvement over the present state of the art. However, in some instances, stakeholders may want to ask questions relevant to cost, quality, or access that cannot be readily answered from what is available in the data base. For example, an employer may find that severity-adjusted posthospital morbidity following CABG surgery is higher for its employees than for the state average. To investigate why, the employer may want to conduct a special survey of employees who have had CABG surgery in the past year to investigate what limitations the employees face in returning to work. Alternatively, a health plan may find that women from a particular geographic area are not receiving prenatal care at the same rate as the rest of the plan's population, despite the apparent availability of providers. To increase the rate, the plan may choose to survey a sample of women in this area to better understand their use of services and their health beliefs. In other words, although an integrated data system that includes clinical data would assist tremendously in the evaluation of costs and quality within and across systems, such appraisals may also raise new questions that may require further study.

Chapter Eight

AN OVERVIEW OF METHODS FOR CONDUCTING SURVEYS

by Lisa Schmidt, Sally C. Morton, Cheryl Damberg, and Elizabeth A. McGlynn

INTRODUCTION

For many questions of interest to health policymakers, data do not exist to answer the questions. In some cases, a survey is the best approach to obtaining needed information (see Chapter Five). The purpose of this chapter is to provide an overview of survey research including

- Designing and conducting surveys;

- Drawing a sample;

- Choosing a mode of survey administration;

- Writing a questionnaire;

- Implementing surveys; and,

- Contracting out survey tasks.

Because of the complexity of this topic, however, we encourage those who are planning to do a survey to obtain a book on survey design and to consult an expert (e.g., a statistician or psychometrician). There are numerous books on survey design to choose from. Weisberg and Bowen (1977) and Moser and Kalton (1971) are two good texts; other references are cited in the Bibliography.

DESIGNING AND CONDUCTING A SURVEY

Before embarking on a survey, it is important to become familiar with all the steps that are needed to properly conduct a survey. Significant costs, both financial and personnel, need to be taken into consideration first. For example, time and resources are required to write the questions, pretest, and revise the questionnaire; train the interviewers; complete the interviews; record the responses; and analyze the data. The major steps required to design and conduct a survey are as follows (adapted from Aday, 1989):

- Determine the type of information to be obtained through the survey;
- Determine the type of study design based on the objectives of the survey;
- Define the survey variables;
- Plan the analysis of the survey data;
- Choose the method of data collection;
- Draw the sample;
- Formulate the questions;
- Format the questionnaire;
- Pretest the questionnaire;
- Monitor and carry out the survey;
- Prepare the data for analysis;
- Implement the analysis of the survey data; and,
- Write a report on the results of the survey.

Survey design is an iterative process that evolves as the decisions are made in response to results occurring at various stages of the process. For example, when pretesting the survey, you may discover that certain questions do not work—your pretest respondents may interpret the question in a different way than you anticipated or they may not understand a question and fail to answer. Therefore, you will have to go back a few steps and reformulate some of your questions and pretest a second time.

A common misstep in survey design is to spend too little time on the first four steps listed above. A *concept key*, which lists the various concepts of interest, the exact variables that will be used to measure those concepts, and the source of those variables, is extremely valuable at the initial stages of planning a survey. Table 8.1 illustrates this approach.

Survey data can be collected in many different ways. The best survey design will depend on the questions to be answered and the study objectives. The first step in survey research is to formulate the questions. For example, if you are interested in how enrollee satisfaction with a health plan varies by age, gender, race, education level, or insurance type (commercial, Medicare, or Medicaid), a one-time (cross-sectional) self-administered survey of a random sample drawn from all the members enrolled in that health plan will be adequate. However, if

Table 8.1

Illustrative Concept Key

Variable	Data Source[a]	Concept Measured				
		Satisfaction	Length of Enrollment	Health Status	Demographics	Insurance Type
Overall satisfaction	S	X				
Rating of access	S	X				
Rating of interpersonal manner	S	X				
Recommend to friends	S	X				
Likelihood of continued enrollment	S	X				
Date of enrollment	A		X			
Date of disenrollment	A		X			
Overall health	S			X		
No. of chronic diseases	A			X		
Age	A, S				X	
Gender	A				X	
Race	S				X	
Education	S				X	
Income	S				X	
Insurer	A					X

[a]S = survey data; A = administrative data.

you want to determine how enrollee satisfaction with the health plan has changed over time, you should do a longitudinal study (e.g., repeat the measurements over time on the same sample). Table 8.2 outlines some of the basic options available in survey design. Each choice will be discussed in more detail below.

Table 8.2

Some Options for Survey Design

Choices	Key Features
Method of sampling	
Probability	Can generalize statistically to the population
Nonprobability	Cannot generalize statistically to the population
Mode of administration	
Mail	Low response rate
Telephone	Moderate response rate
Face-to-face	High response rate
Time period addressed	
Cross-sectional	Measures at one point in time; population may be different in subsequent years (i.e., if survey is repeated)
Longitudinal	Tracks changes over time (multiple measures of the same population)

SAMPLING THE STUDY POPULATION

Methods of Sampling

When conducting a survey, it is not necessary to survey the entire population you are interested in studying—for example, all persons enrolled in a particular health plan or all patients admitted to a particular hospital. Statistical methods can be employed to understand how data from a *sample* of the population of interest can be used to generalize to the whole population. If the respondents are randomly sampled, the results based on the sample are likely to be representative of the entire population. Statistical methods will also help you quantify the extent to which the use of a sample introduces uncertainty into your results.

A key, and sometimes overlooked, step is constructing the *sampling frame*. This is the population of interest from which a sample will be drawn. Research is frequently conducted in managed care organizations and on the Medicare population because the sampling frame is more easily constructed because the entire population is known. Research at the community or state level is more difficult because the eligible population is not completely known. A clear identification of the population is essential for sampling methods to be properly applied.

The goal in drawing a sample is to select a group of individuals that is representative of all individuals in the population. In thinking about whom to survey, there are various methods you could use to draw a sample. The decision about which method to use depends on the questions being asked and your budget.

Sampling methods can be classified into two categories:

- Probability; and
- Nonprobability.

In *probability sampling* (sometimes called random sampling), each person in the population being studied has a known chance of being included in the sample. The simplest type of probability sample is a simple random sample in which every member of the population has an equal probability of being sampled. Knowing the probability with which each member of the population is sampled allows you to estimate the unknown result for the entire population based on the data obtained from those who were sampled. The precision of the estimate can be calculated using well-developed statistical methods. The randomness of your sampling procedure ensures that your sample represents the population in an unbiased way.

In *nonprobability sampling*, however, the chance of any particular individual being selected is not known; therefore, the results of the sample cannot be generalized to the larger population of interest. Generalizations that are drawn have no statistical foundation, such as is necessary for measuring the accuracy of the generalization. If the sample is also not drawn randomly, the results may also be biased.

A probability sample is the preferred approach because it limits the potential for bias resulting from the sampling design and allows you to quantify the accuracy of your results. A nonprobability sample is rarely justifiable with the possible exception of developmental work.

It is important to distinguish sampling design decisions from what actually occurs when that design is implemented. Any result for a population based on a random sample will contain some error. The error can be divided into two components: sampling error and bias. Sampling error results because you have randomly sampled only a subset of individuals. Sampling error can be decreased by increasing your sample size, and, in fact, sampling error decreases proportional to the square root of the sample size. Thus, if you quadruple your sample size, you halve your sampling error.

Bias, which is a systematic tendency to overestimate or underestimate the result you are interested in, can be introduced if the sample that answers the survey is not completely random. This is a common problem in surveys. Bias can be decreased only by changing the way you draw your sample or through study procedures designed to minimize anticipated problems. For example, if poor people are less likely to respond because you are conducting a telephone survey and poor people are less likely to have telephones, you may have to add face-to-face interviews for a subsample of poor individuals to reduce your nonresponse bias. Any survey with low response rates (e.g., less than 80 percent) is likely to suffer from bias. Thus, even though your design is an unbiased random sample, theoretically, the implementation of that design may introduce bias. Methods for addressing these sorts of problems are discussed in Chapter Six.

There are several ways to conduct both probability and nonprobability sampling. These approaches are defined briefly in Table 8.3.

Choosing a Sample Size

Sample size is very important because it can affect the probability that you will see an effect in your data; for example, that the satisfaction of enrollees in one health plan is different from that in another health plan, if indeed such a difference exists. This probability is known as statistical *power*. In addition, having a

Table 8.3

Some Common Approaches to Sampling

Sampling Approach	Description
	Probability
Simple random sampling	A sampling method in which every person in the population of interest has a known and equal chance of being selected. One way to draw a simple random sample is to use a random number generator to select people. Another approach is to draw a systematic random sample. A random person between the first and the nth person on a list of the population is chosen as the first person sampled, and then every nth person thereafter is chosen. For example, if a sample of 100 is desired from a total population of 1,000, then the sampling interval n would be determined by dividing the total sample population by the desired sample size (e.g., 1,000 ÷ 100 = 10). If the population list is randomly ordered, a systematic random sample is equivalent to a simple random sample. However, bias can be inadvertently introduced if the population list is arranged in some order related to the study question (e.g., by insurance type).
Stratified sampling	This method draws random samples from mutually exclusive and exhaustive subgroups ("strata") of the population of interest (i.e., nonoverlapping subgroups that together contain the entire population). Examples of strata include geographic region, type of hospital (public vs. private), demographic characteristics such as gender, and diagnoses. This approach can improve the sample's accuracy but is generally more expensive than a simple random sample. It also allows estimation for each stratum individually, for example, estimating the quality of care for public hospitals, which may be a secondary goal of a hospital care survey. In fact, oversampling, that is, drawing a larger proportion of the sample from a particular stratum than the proportion of the population as a whole that exists in that stratum, may be done to improve the precision of that particular stratum's estimate and is often used when the number of persons randomly sampled would be too small for separate analysis.
Cluster sampling	A method by which individuals are selected through a hierarchical process. This approach, which takes advantage of existing groupings of populations, is often used to reduce survey costs. For example, one may be interested in comparing the outcomes of bypass surgery in different hospitals in the state. The first step is to sample hospitals (clusters) that represent strata of interest (public vs. private, large vs. small, north vs. south). Next, within each hospital a random sample of patients who had bypass surgery is selected. This method is less costly than randomly sampling patients across all hospitals, which would require enlisting many more hospitals into the study. However, because patients within the same hospital may have similar experiences because of hospital policy, staffing, location, facilities, or other factors, a cluster sample is not as informative as a simple random sample of the same number of patients. You may not be able to disentangle the result from the factors that are correlated with the result.
	Nonprobability
Convenience sampling	Individuals are selected in a way that is easy for the researcher, which means that the likelihood of any participant being in the sample is unknown and deliberately not random. For example, a survey might be done on patients who present for care in a single doctor's office. This method is prone to bias and should only be used for exploratory work (e.g., developing a survey).

Table 8.3 (continued)

Sampling Approach	Description
Quota sampling	This method sets a predetermined number of persons to be included based on certain characteristics such as geographic location, gender, age, or race/ethnicity. Often quotas are established to represent the known distributions in the population. For example, you may want a sample of 100 persons to include 20 blacks. The quota approach would continue to seek respondents until 20 blacks were included. This group may differ from both the other 80 in the survey and from the population they were selected to represent. This approach is generally not recommended because it tends to introduce bias into the sample.
Purposive sampling	In this method, someone uses his or her own judgment about which respondents to choose for the sample. The advantage of this method is that skill and prior knowledge can be used to choose the respondents. This method is also used sometimes when data systems are inadequate for identifying the population of interest (e.g., those with an outpatient diagnosis of asthma). However, this approach introduces obvious bias into the sample as the person doing the choosing may select only those who are likely to prove a particular study hypothesis.

sufficient sample size is important for drawing precise conclusions from your survey.

Power and precision calculations to determine what sample size is necessary are based on minimizing sampling error. In addition, you must be concerned about bias. For example, it is rare for everyone selected in your sample to agree to participate. Thus, estimating the proportion of people who will not respond is important so that you have an adequate final sample size to ensure that the sampling error is acceptable. Even more important is the fact that nonrespondents may differ from respondents, and ignoring nonresponse could bias your results.

Choosing the appropriate sample size depends on the nature of the population and the purpose of the study. If your entire population is small, say 10 to 12 individuals, it is probably wise to sample 100 percent of the population. In most cases, however, the population of interest is relatively large (e.g., entire groups of health plan enrollees or all practicing physicians in a health plan) so sampling is appropriate. A common oversight is failure to calculate sample sizes needed for analyses of subgroups (e.g., white vs. nonwhite, male vs. female, or low income vs. high income). To avoid undersampling, the subgroups you wish to study should be identified and required sample sizes should be estimated for those groups before collecting data. You might need to take into account differential response rates among subgroups in determining the number to be sampled.

As an example, say you surveyed 100 enrollees in your health plan to determine their satisfaction with the health services they have received. After collecting the data, you decide you want to see if satisfaction varies by insurance status (e.g., commercial, Medicare, or Medicaid). After categorizing the respondents by insurance status, you determine that your sample contains 85 commercial enrollees, 10 Medicare enrollees, and 5 Medicaid enrollees. Unfortunately, you did not survey enough Medicare and Medicaid enrollees to do any separate analyses on these populations. This example reinforces the importance of thinking through how your data will be subdivided during data analysis (e.g., into age categories, race/ethnic groups, or educational levels) before deciding upon your sample to ensure an adequate sample size for each subdivision.

Chapter Six discusses these issues in more detail and includes precision and power calculations to determine required sample size. You should consult with a statistician to determine the appropriate sample size for your survey.

MODES OF SURVEY ADMINISTRATION

Surveys can be administered in a variety of ways, including by telephone, mail (self-administered), or interviewer-administered (face-to-face). All surveys have been enhanced by computer-assisted data-gathering methods. Computer-assisted telephone interviewing (CATI) is the most well-developed and widely used computerized mode of data gathering. Computer-assisted personal interviewing (CAPI) and computerized self-administered questionnaires (CSAQ) are in less widespread use.

The choice of method for administering the survey is often based on an evaluation of the various tradeoffs associated with each approach. Tradeoffs typically pertain to cost, accuracy, types of questions that can be asked, and the ease of conducting the survey. Table 8.4 provides a simple comparison between the three modes of survey administration. In addition, the basic features of the three methods are briefly described. It is common for these methods to be used in combination to increase response rates and minimize bias resulting from nonresponse among subgroups in the population.

Self-administered *mail surveys* are among the most common methods for collecting data and are easy to conduct; however, they typically have low response rates on a single mailing. Mail surveys are generally sent to a respondent with a cover letter and instructions to return the survey by a certain date. Follow-up reminders, either by mail or telephone, and participation incentives (e.g., cash or gift certificates) are usually required to obtain an adequate response rate. Mail surveys should generally be shorter than similar surveys conducted by telephone or face-to-face to achieve similar response rates. It is difficult to

Table 8.4

Comparison of Interviewing Methods

Feature	Interview Method		
	Mail	Telephone	Face-to-Face
Cost per completed interview	Low—depends on postage rate and use of incentives	Medium—depends on toll charges, which increase with distance from calling location	High—requires travel time and costs and greater interviewer training and skill
Cost of random sampling	Inexpensive, but follow-up costs can be high to achieve acceptable response rates	Moderately expensive; varies with accuracy of telephone numbers	Expensive—respondents may be spread over a large geographic area
Response rate[a]	Typically low (< 50 percent)	Moderate (60 to 70 percent)	High (80 percent or greater)
Potential length of survey	Short (20 to 30 minutes)	Short (20 to 40 minutes)	Long (one hour)

SOURCE: Adapted from Weisberg and Bowen (1977).

[a]For a discussion of bias resulting from response rate, see Chapter Six.

define a maximum length for a questionnaire; however, Dillman (1978) reports that going beyond 12 pages seems almost certain to affect response rate. Although there is a widely held perception that self-administered mail surveys are relatively low cost, the cost of conducting such surveys is highly variable depending on the methods used to obtain the highest possible response rate (telephone follow-up, repeating mailings, or incentives). Nonresponse bias is a concern in mail surveys.

Low response rates can be a concern if people who did respond to the survey differ from those who did not respond along the dimensions you are measuring (e.g., satisfaction with care). If respondents differ from nonrespondents, the conclusions that you draw from the survey may be biased. For example, health plan enrollees who are satisfied with the care they received may be less likely to respond to a mailed questionnaire than those who are dissatisfied. Analyzing a survey with this response pattern might lead you to conclude that the majority of enrollees are dissatisfied with care. If you based your conclusions on information provided largely by dissatisfied respondents and do not capture information from satisfied customers, you may overstate the level of dissatisfaction among health plan enrollees. See Chapter Six for a discussion of biases.

Interviewer-administered *telephone surveys* are also relatively easy to conduct and typically have higher response rates than mail surveys. Telephone surveys can be done more quickly than mail surveys because you do not have to wait for receipt and return of questionnaires. They often have high rates of response and therefore may be worth the additional cost, depending on the issue of interest and your budget. Telephone surveys can typically be longer than mail questionnaires but shorter than face-to-face interviews. Approximately 5 percent of respondents who begin a telephone interview terminate it before completion (Bailey, 1987), but this varies widely depending on the way the sample was identified, the nature of the survey, and the skill of the interviewer. Telephone interviews also require interviewer training, which can increase costs. Biased results can occur with telephone surveys, however, if nonresponse results from not being able to reach the person you want to interview (e.g., they are not home when you call) or because the individual elects not to respond. In addition, bias can be introduced if the people who have a telephone and complete the survey are different from those you cannot interview because they do not have a telephone. If you believe that income may be an important factor (e.g., access to medical care) in your results, then this type of bias is particularly problematic.

Face-to-face interviewer-administered surveys are the most costly mode of administration; however, the advantages of this method are high response rates. Bailey (1987) reports that very few face-to-face respondents will terminate interviews once they have begun. Also, this method of survey typically permits the collection of larger amounts of information because the length of the interview can typically be longer than that of mailed questionnaires or telephone interviews. One possible disadvantage of this survey method is that individuals may be more reluctant to answer questions they perceive as embarrassing or sensitive (e.g., income or sexual practices). This may introduce bias into your results if the respondents do not answer the questions truthfully. Also, the interviewer may introduce bias into the results if he or she encourages (either explicitly through directions or implicitly through body language) a person to respond in a particular way. More extensive training is required of face-to-face interviewers than telephone interviewers to avoid these potential sources of bias.

CROSS-SECTIONAL, LONGITUDINAL, AND REPEATED CROSS-SECTIONAL DESIGNS

The three most common types of survey designs are cross-sectional, longitudinal, and repeated cross-sectional. In cross-sectional surveys, data are collected at one point in time from a sample representative of the population you are interested in surveying. These surveys can be used for descriptive purposes and for determining the relationships between variables at the time of the study.

For example, a patient satisfaction questionnaire can be used to determine satisfaction with a health plan at a particular time. In addition, if health status questions were asked in the survey, statistical analysis could be conducted to determine the relationship between patient satisfaction and health status.

Longitudinal surveys are conducted at different points in time on the same population and can be used to explain how the concept being measured (e.g., patient satisfaction) changes over time. If you wish to study changes over time for a defined group, you will have to conduct a longitudinal study. In the third approach, repeated cross-sectional survey, you repeat the same questionnaire at regular intervals on a new sample drawn from the same population (e.g., health plan members enrolled for a full year). The main difference between the longitudinal and repeated cross-section is the people in the sample. The longitudinal design has the advantage of using the same respondents so that changes in results can be interpreted as time changes. In repeated cross-sections, it may be difficult to distinguish between time trends and sample differences. On the other hand, longitudinal panels are subject to attrition over time (e.g., people may die or move), and over several years this may have the same effect—the people enrolled in the longitudinal panel for multiple years are different from those who were represented at the beginning of the study.

The selection of design depends on the question you are trying to answer and the effect of different design features on the interpretability of the results. In addition, for obvious reasons, longitudinal studies are much more expensive than cross-sectional surveys; therefore, the size of your budget may affect the type of survey design you choose.

CONTENT OF THE SURVEY

Up to this point, we have discussed the design of the survey and whom to survey. We will now discuss *what questions* to ask in the survey. Specifically, we will focus on how the questions should be worded, what response choices should be made available to the respondents, and in what sequence the questions should be asked. All of these issues are important to consider when writing the questionnaire.

Preliminary Steps in Choosing Survey Questions

You should keep five issues in mind before beginning to write your survey questions. They are as follows (adapted from Aday, 1989):

1. The principal research question, study objectives, and hypotheses should guide the selection of questions for the survey.

Each question in the survey should be related to your research question or be an important control variable. Before including a question, think about how the results will be analyzed. If you cannot determine how the data will be used, then do not include it. The tradeoffs of including irrelevant questions could be lower response rates, because the questionnaire becomes too long, or missing data, because the respondent does not see the relevance of particular questions and refuses to answer them.

2. Do not try to reinvent the wheel.

Look for other studies that have dealt with similar topics. Review the questionnaires and articles that summarize the methods and results of those studies. Determine whether formal tests of the validity and reliability of specific questions or scales have been conducted. It is important to determine whether there were methodological problems with the questions. For example, were there high rates of missing values because of confusing wording or embarrassing questions? If possible, it may be useful to talk to the person who designed the questions to determine how well the questions worked in their survey and what they would do differently if they could do the survey over again.

3. Consider the best way to ask a particular type of question.

Ask yourself whether the questions are about factual and objective characteristics or behaviors, nonfactual and subjective attitudes or perceptions, or indicators of health status. People may be better able to answer some questions than others. For example, people are generally not able to accurately report their insurance coverage; this information might be better obtained from an objective source if correctly classifying people by insurance type is important. On the other hand, you might be interested in people's perception of the generosity of their insurance if you believe that is likely to predict health service use.

4. Consider the extent to which the mode of questionnaire administration will affect responses to questions in a survey.

Verbal and visual cues provided by the interviewer in a face-to-face interview may influence the response to a question. In telephone interviews, verbal communication (the way the question is asked or voice inflection) may influence the way a respondent answers a question. In self-administered questionnaires, the main influence is visual (as the respondent reads the question); the way the questions are written, the question order, and the type of answer choices provided can affect answers to a question. For example, sensitive topics (such as sexual practices) might be more accurately reported in a self-administered mail survey than in face-to-face interviews.

5. **Keep in mind the types of errors that can arise at each stage in developing survey questions and the approaches to minimizing or eliminating such errors.**

Each mode of questionnaire administration is prone to different errors. We advise you to consult experts or textbooks related to the type of questionnaire you are implementing to understand how to minimize errors. Some textbook suggestions are Sudman and Bradburn (1982) and Dillman (1978).

Questionnaire Construction

It would be impossible in this chapter to discuss in detail all the important aspects of questionnaire design. What follows is a checklist of helpful hints. We encourage you to seek assistance from the textbooks listed above or to consult with an expert in survey research.

Wording of Questions. Do not include *double-barreled questions*, that is, two or more questions in one. If you write questions with "*or*" or "*and*" in them, check to see if they contain two questions with only one answer expected. For example, "Do you believe that AIDS can be transmitted by shaking hands with or by drinking out of the same glass as a person with AIDS?" This question really asks about an individual's opinion about two different modes of HIV transmission. This question should be divided into two separate questions.

Avoid ambiguous questions in which the words themselves are vague or the meaning of the word may be known only to highly educated persons. In addition, avoid words that may mean different things to people living in different geographic areas, age groups, or cultures. An example of an ambiguously worded question might be, "In which social class do your parents belong: upper, upper middle, middle, lower middle or lower class?" One ambiguous word here is "belong." Some people may interpret it as the class they are *currently* in; others may interpret it as the class they *deserve* to be in or *ought* to be in. In addition, categories such as "upper" and "upper middle" are ambiguous, and the determinants of social class may vary by population groups. There is no clear cutoff between the responses. For this question, it might be better to ask about household income.

Level of wording is important. Questions should be written for the educational level of the population you are surveying. Many respondents are embarrassed to admit they do not understand a word and will give any answer instead of asking for clarification of the word. Cognitive testing is one way to determine if the level of question wording is too high. Cognitive testing can be conducted in several ways. One approach is to have an individual complete a questionnaire and then interview them about what they thought about in answering the question. This may provide some insight into whether respondents are interpreting the question as you intended. If the population you are studying uses slang or colloquialisms, be sure you use those terms in your questionnaire so that the respondents will understand the questions. One way to discover slang terms is through focus groups. A focus group is a small, generally convenience sample of people who are similar to those who will be studied who are led through a discussion of a topic by a skilled facilitator following a pre-established protocol. If you are surveying a group of individuals with disabilities, you could conduct a focus group of people with disabilities to learn how they refer to some of their services. For example, many persons with disabilities have someone come into their home to help them with daily activities such as bathing, dressing, cooking, and cleaning. We may refer to the person who comes into the disabled person's home as an "assistant" but many persons with disabilities refer to that person as their "provider" or "choreworker" or "home care aide."

Questions should not be leading. They should be carefully structured to minimize the probability of biasing the respondent's answer by suggesting that there is a correct or preferred response. Questions should be asked in a neutral form, such as, "Do you think that smoking is harmful to your health?" rather than, "The majority of physicians feel that smoking is harmful to your health, do you agree?"

Avoid sensitive or threatening questions. Questions related to sensitive topics such as sex, drug use, or suicide are prone to normative answers—respondents may give answers that are consistent with norms of society, even though they may be false. There are several ways to encourage a respondent to answer a sensitive question truthfully even if that answer is not socially desirable. First, phrase questions in a way that assumes that he or she engages in that behavior but provide a response that would force him or her to deny it. For example, instead of asking "Do you use marijuana? Yes or No. If yes how often?" ask "How frequently do you use marijuana: every day, once a week, once a month, never?" Second, word the question so as to presume that there is no consensus regarding the norm. For example, "Some doctors feel that drinking is harmful and others feel it is beneficial: What do you think?" Third, word the question so that the behavior does not seem deviant. For example, when asking about drug use ask "Many people have tried marijuana at one time or another, have you?"

Response Categories. Wording of the question is only part of the art of questionnaire construction. Careful attention must be given to the response categories provided. There is generally a distinction made between *open-ended* and *closed-ended* questions. Open-ended questions are those for which response categories are not specified; closed-ended questions require respondents to select from predetermined responses. In general, open-ended questions are used only in developmental work because of difficulty in interpretation and coding. Table 8.5 lists advantages and disadvantages of each type of question.

In closed-ended questions, the number of response categories is an important consideration. Answer categories for a nominal variable (discrete categories that cannot be ranked) must be mutually exclusive (only one correct category for each respondent) and exhaustive (a category for every respondent). If there are many possible categories, but only a handful of common responses, you may print the common categories and provide a response of "other." The "other" category provides minimal information to the researcher but allows all respondents to answer. An example of a nominal variable is race. The answer categories for the variable race could be an exhaustive list of all possible races or, as is more commonly done, a list of several race categories with an "other" category for those who do not describe themselves as belonging to one of the categories listed. For example:

Which category best describes your race? Are you . . .

1) Asian/Pacific Islander
2) Black
3) Hispanic
4) White
5) Other

Many questionnaire items are opinion or attitude questions in which the answers are ordinal (discrete categories that can be rank-ordered). The categories may be subjective and are defined by the researcher. For example:

How would you rate the overall quality of health services you received?

1) Excellent
2) Very good
3) Good
4) Fair
5) Poor

In this case, the responses are ordered with "excellent" representing the highest overall quality of services and "poor" representing the lowest overall quality of services.

Table 8.5

Advantages and Disadvantages of Closed-Ended and Open-Ended Questions

Advantages	Disadvantages
Closed-Ended	
Produces standard answers that can be compared from person to person	It is easy for a respondent who does not know the answer or has no opinion to guess or answer randomly
Answers can often be coded directly from the questionnaire and analyzed directly saving time and money	The appropriate response category may not be provided or is not provided in sufficient detail
Respondent is often clearer about the meaning of the question based on the responses provided	Too many answer categories can lead to rereading or repeating of categories resulting in lengthier and costlier interviews
Answers tend to be more complete and a minimum of irrelevant responses are received	Differences in interpretation of the question may go undetected
Burden is reduced because respondent merely has to choose a category	True variability in answers among respondents may be eliminated by forced-choice responses
	Errors in choice of response if, for example, a respondent circles choice 2 but meant to circle 3
Open-Ended	
Useful when all of the possible answer categories are not known	May lead to collection of worthless, irrelevant, or uninterpretable information
Allows the respondent to answer adequately, in all the detail he or she likes and to clarify his or her answer	Data are not standardized from person to person, making coding comparison or statistical analyses difficult
Preferable for complex issues that cannot be condensed into a few small categories	Requires superior writing or speaking skills, ability to articulate one's feelings, and generally higher education level than closed-ended questions
Allows for more creativity and self-expression by the respondent	Questions may be too general, requiring use of probes or more specific follow-up questions administered by the interviewer, thus not acceptable for mail or self-administered questionnaires
	Requires more time and effort of respondent leading to a higher nonresponse rate
	May introduce coding errors by interviewer (for oral responses) or coder (for written)

The researcher may choose to provide a category for those who have no opinion or for whom the question does not apply. There is a tradeoff, however, in deciding whether to provide these as response categories. If "don't know" or "does not apply" categories are not provided, the respondent is forced to choose one of the answers or to leave the question blank. The response may be inaccurate if the answer is chosen at random and the respondent has no opinion or the question does not apply to him or her. On the other hand, including the "don't know" or "does not apply" categories provides an easy opportunity for the respondent to avoid thinking about the question and simply choose one of these categories; this could lead to inaccuracies in the data. When completing your data analysis, these responses are usually counted as "missing values" and will affect the size of your sample. If this was not anticipated in the power calculation, it may affect the statistical significance and the results of your study. See Chapter Six for more information on such data analysis issues.

Question Order

When combining questions to form the final questionnaire, you must decide how many questions to include and in which order to present them. In general, questions should be put in the following order (Bailey, 1987):

1. **Put sensitive questions and open-ended questions late in the questionnaire, unless critical to study purpose.**

If sensitive questions are encountered first, the respondent may choose not to continue with the questionnaire. It they are last, then at least all the nonsensitive questions are already answered, even if the respondent refuses to answer the sensitive questions. The exception is when the sensitive questions are the key content for the study. You may want to ensure that partial responses include these questions. Open-ended questions should also be placed toward the end of the questionnaire because they generally require more thought and time. If respondents spend a great deal of time on open-ended questions in the beginning, they may not finish the rest of the questionnaire. When respondents fail to complete the entire questionnaire, your sample size for the unanswered questions is reduced because those data must be treated as missing.

2. **Ask easy-to-answer questions first.**

The first question should be easy to answer, should not be threatening to the respondent, and should have distinct answer categories. In addition, it should be about a fact rather than an opinion. For example, a good question to begin with is gender or age.

3. Ask information needed for subsequent questions, first.

It is often helpful to first elicit information that will be useful to answering sub-sequent questions. For example, if asking a question about family members, it might be helpful to ask about family size or household first so the respondent has the right frame of reference in answering questions about the family. Com-puterized survey tools can make use of these answers either by "filling" infor-mation into later questions or by "branching" people into only those questions that apply to them. For example, if you were surveying the Medicare popula-tion about use of preventive services you could use answers to the gender ques-tion to branch only men into questions about screening for prostate cancer and women into questions about screening for breast cancer.

4. Place questions in logical order.

Place all questions about a given topic together. For example, ask all questions regarding employment history or health service use together and do not jump back and forth between them. Also, place questions in a logical time sequence. For example, when asking questions about employment history, you will make it easier for the respondent to reply in a sequence, either first job to present job or present job back to first job. Maintaining the same time frame throughout a questionnaire, where appropriate, will also minimize respondent confusion.

5. Avoid establishing a response set.

A response set is a tendency to reply to items in the same way, regardless of the question's content or the correct answer. For example, if statements are phrased so that agreement is always the preferred response, a respondent may just circle the same response all the way down a series of questions without even reading the questions. This decreases real variability in responses. One way to avoid this is to vary the question or answer format from question to question. The disadvantages to this are that the respondent's train of thought might be broken or he or she may get confused.

6. Separate reliability-check questions pairs.

Pairs of questions, one stated positively and one negatively, are often used to check reliability. For example, at one point in the questionnaire you might ask "Abortion should be legalized (agree/disagree)" and a later point ask "Abortion should not be legalized (agree/disagree)." Such question pairs will enable you to detect unreliable questions and remove them from the data analysis.

7. Vary questions by length and type.

Vary question format, response format, length, and open and closed-ended questions. This may help maintain respondent interest, but it also could make the questionnaire more difficult to answer.

IMPLEMENTING THE SURVEY

Introduction and Instruction

Every questionnaire, whether mailed, telephone, or face-to-face interview, should have an introductory statement. This statement will serve to introduce the purpose of the survey to the respondent, explain why it is important, and reassure the respondent that his or her responses will not be revealed to others. It should

- Identify the persons or organizations conducting the survey;

- Tell why the survey is important and why the respondent should be willing to complete it;

- Assure the respondent that there are no right or wrong answers; and,

- Tell the respondent what to expect regarding confidentiality.

It is usually necessary to include instructions for respondents in a mailed self-administered questionnaire. If the interview is done by telephone or in person, the interviewer can both provide instructions and answer questions to make sure the respondent understands what is expected. Mailed questionnaires are usually limited to questions that require only simple instructions for answering, since the respondent will not have access to anyone to ask questions. Very often in mailed questionnaires, the instructions for answering will be repeated with each individual question. For example (Bailey, 1987):

The doctor can't help you keep your child from getting sick with TB if it runs in your family (CIRCLE ONE)

Strongly agree	 1
Agree	 2
Disagree	 3
Strongly disagree	 4

In addition to providing instructions with each question, general instructions can be included at the beginning of the questionnaire. For example (Bailey, 1987):

GENERAL INSTRUCTIONS: Most of the questions ask you only to circle the number that represents the answer of your choice. For example:

Often   1
Sometimes   2
Rarely   3
Never   4

Some questions ask you to fill in an appropriate number, word, or phrase on the line provided: _____ years.

Some questions are not to be answered by everyone. For example:

Yes   1
No   . . . . 2 (SKIP TO Q #5)

The person who answers "yes" would continue to the next question. The person who answers "no" would skip to question #5. Skip patterns can be confusing in self-administered surveys, resulting in some inconsistent responses.

There really are no general rules for writing instructions except to remember that they *are* necessary and they must be clear and easy to follow. Many instructions will be formulated as you write the questionnaire. In addition, you will identify areas that need clarification by instructions during the pretest.

Maximizing Response Rates

The importance of response rates cannot be overemphasized. What you can reasonably conclude from a survey is dependent on the rate of response you are able to obtain. Low response rates almost certainly mean that the results are biased even if the demographic distribution reflects that of the overall population. This is because nonrespondents are very likely to hold different opinions or have had different experiences than those who did respond. Response rates vary by mode of survey administration as discussed above and are calculated as follows:

$$\text{Response rate} = \frac{\text{number of completed questionnaires}}{\text{number of eligible sampled units}} \times 100$$

Although in many cases the extent of the differences between respondents and nonrespondents cannot be determined, any opportunity to quantify the difference should be taken. For example, in face-to-face or telephone interviews, the interviewer may be able to ask the individual why he or she does not wish to respond and may even be able to obtain some demographic information (e.g., age or gender). In mail questionnaires, however, because there is no personal contact between the respondent and the researcher, there is usually no way to determine any personal characteristics of the nonrespondent. However, you may be able to obtain some from the information that generated the sampling frame or list of the population from which you sampled, or by following up with a telephone call to solicit demographic information (a nonresponse survey).

Depending on whether the survey is face-to-face, by telephone, or by mail, there are many ways in which response rates can be enhanced. In general, Dillman (1978) recommends:

1. *Rewarding* the respondent by

- Showing positive regard;
- Giving verbal appreciation;
- Offering tangible rewards; and,
- Making the questionnaire interesting.

Examples of rewards include: taking the time to explain to someone that they are part of a carefully selected sample and that their response is needed if the study is to be successful; personalizing questionnaires by using real signatures, individual salutations, and individually typed letters; and, providing incentives such as cash, gift certificates, or other tangible items such as pencils or a mug.

2. *Reducing costs* to the respondent by

- Making the task as brief as possible;
- Reducing the physical and mental effort that is required;
- Eliminating chances for embarrassment; and,
- Eliminating any direct monetary cost to the respondent.

In mail or other self-administered surveys, it is important not to make questionnaires look overwhelming. For example, reducing the number of pages and using an appropriate font size (not too small) can help increase response rate by decreasing the respondent's expectation of the amount of time it will take to complete. In addition, furnishing a stamped, self-addressed return envelope will help increase response rates. In telephone or face-to-face interviews, assuring the respondent that the questionnaire will take only a short time will encourage the respondent to continue.

3. *Establishing trust* by

- Providing a token of appreciation in advance; and,
- Identifying with a known organization that has legitimacy to the respondent.

A financial incentive (e.g., a $5 bill or check enclosed with the mailed survey) may help establish trust between the respondent and the researcher by assuring the respondent that the researcher has good faith that the questionnaire/interview will be completed. However, larger monetary incentives do not always lead to higher response rates and at least some level may be seen by the respondent as coercive. Providing the incentive before the completion of the questionnaire is more effective than promising to send it after the survey is returned. Another way to establish trust is to make sure that the survey is identified with a known organization. For example, reference to a local college, university, or foundation may lead the respondent to complete the questionnaire if they have received prior benefits from that organization. When physicians are respondents, endorsement by a specialty society or the local medical society may be helpful.

Another important activity that can substantially increase response rates is following up with postcards or telephone calls. In mail surveys, usually after the initial mailing, a response rate of approximately 25 percent can be expected. However, with a second mailing and a reminder postcard, a response rate of 50 percent or more can be expected. In addition, telephone reminders can be used for mailed questionnaires if phone numbers are known. For telephone interviews, it is common to make at least three attempts to contact the respondent before classifying the individual as a nonrespondent.

WHO SHOULD ADMINISTER THE SURVEY?

Conducting a survey is a very large task. As indicated in this chapter, there is more to a survey than simply sending out a questionnaire and tallying up responses. Considerable staff time, resources, and expertise are required. If you decide that a survey is the best way for you to get the information you need, there are many resources you should consult if you need help in completing your survey. In addition, there are many organizations you can contract with to conduct almost any aspect of a survey.

For example, unless you have a printing department in your organization, you will probably want to contract out the job of printing your questionnaire. If you are doing a mail questionnaire, you can contract with an organization to print the mailing labels, stuff the envelopes, and mail the questionnaire. In telephone surveys, you can contract out the telephone interviewing to a firm that has the staff and equipment to do large-scale telephone interviewing. For any type of survey, you can contract out data entry. Almost any job related to surveying can be contracted out depending on your needs and budget. The *American Association of Public Opinion Researchers* directory is a good place to start to locate firms that can help you with some of your surveying tasks. Contracting does not guarantee that the survey will be conducted as suggested here. The quality of firms varies considerably and careful attention to design and implementation is essential to ensuring that the ultimate product is useful.

How do you know if you should contract out some of the tasks required to conduct a survey? The first thing you need to do is evaluate your staff time, resources, and expertise. Ask yourself the following questions:

- How much staff time can you devote to the development and implementation of the survey and the analysis of results?

- What is your budget?

- What is the most efficient way to use your budget?

- Will your organization allow you to contract with another organization?

- What expertise do each of your staff members have?

- Do you have time to go through a bidding process, if necessary, to contract out services with another organization?

Basically, the decision rests on how large a survey you are conducting and how much of your staff resources you can devote to each of the required tasks. For example, it may be worth the money to contract out telephone interviewing to free up your staff time for other projects. Another source of help may be volunteers who can complete such tasks as stuffing envelopes and mailing out follow-up reminder notices.

If you do decide to contract out services, you should consider obtaining bids from at least three companies. In obtaining bids, you should develop a list of specifications that you wish the companies to bid on. Specifications are basically a list of tasks from which companies will base their bids. It is important that the specifications be clearly defined and detailed so that you can compare bids across different companies. For example, if you are requesting bids on the costs of mailing out 1,000 questionnaires, you should specify each step involved in that process. The specifications would include printing 1,000 mailing labels; folding, stuffing, and sealing 1,000 envelopes; affixing mailing labels and stamps to 1,000 envelopes; and delivering the envelopes to the post office. Although this may seem too detailed, it is important that each company bid on exactly the same tasks to enable you to compare all the bids.

Again, how many survey tasks you should do in-house and how many you should contract out depends on your resources and your priorities.

Chapter Nine

AN OVERVIEW OF RISK ADJUSTMENT

by June O'Leary, Emmett B. Keeler, Cheryl Damberg, and Eve A. Kerr

INTRODUCTION

Risk or severity adjustment is a method used to account for differences in patient characteristics (e.g., age, income, and type of illness needing treatment) likely to affect the outcomes of care (e.g., death, physical functioning, resource utilization, and cost), *independent* of the actual medical treatment given. In this chapter, risk adjustment will be categorized by its two distinct applications:

1. Adjustment by patient characteristics to *predict the amount and cost of care* that an individual would use with an average provider; and

2. Adjustment by patient characteristics in *comparing health outcomes* (e.g., death and disability) after medical intervention.

In the rest of this chapter, the term *risk adjustment* is used when referring to use or cost of care, whereas the term *severity adjustment* is used when referring to health outcomes. This terminology is not consistently used in the literature, but we chose to make this distinction to clarify the different applications. This chapter is meant to serve as an overview of the topics of risk and severity adjustment. Because the techniques and models (often called systems) available to conduct severity or risk adjustment are complex, the reader is encouraged to obtain the related citations referenced in this chapter.

In addition, we recommend that any analyst who plans to use severity adjustment for comparing health outcomes or risk adjustment for predicting cost and resource utilization also read Chapter Five (Description of Data Sources and Related Issues), Chapter Six (General Analysis Issues), and Chapter Seven (Developing and Using a Clinical Information System).

This chapter will consider risk adjustment and then severity adjustment. For each topic we address:

- What is risk/severity adjustment?

- Why is risk/severity adjustment important?

- When and how is risk/severity adjustment used?

- How is an existing risk-adjustment or severity-adjustment system evaluated?

WHAT IS RISK ADJUSTMENT?

Risk adjustment is a technique to account for differences in the characteristics of an individual that are likely to affect the person's use of medical services and health care spending. Adjusting for differences in risks allows health plans and providers to get paid more appropriately for patients relative to the amount of services they are expected to need.

Risk adjustment typically begins by identifying characteristics that are associated with costs. Data that contain these characteristics and annual costs are analyzed to determine the weights that explain the average amount spent on care by individuals with different characteristics. Subsequently, this weighting scheme or risk-adjustment formula will be used prospectively to predict the amount that individuals or families with any set of specified characteristics will spend in an average year with an average set of providers. Analysts can select from a number of previously developed risk-adjustment systems or try to develop their own.

WHAT FACTORS SHOULD BE CONSIDERED FOR RISK ADJUSTMENT?

To risk-adjust premiums, capitation rates, or payments, we start by identifying factors that are predictive of differences in costs. These factors are called *risk adjusters.* Examples of risk adjusters that have been shown to affect the cost of providing care are described in Table 9.1.

Not all risk adjusters are available from every data source discussed in Chapter Five. Some are relatively easy to access but others are not. The analyst may have to extract information from more than one data source or choose the single best source until clinical information systems are more widely available. Table 9.2 provides some examples of common risk adjusters and the data sources where they may be found.

Table 9.1

Risk-Adjuster Categories and Examples

Category	Examples
Demographic characteristics	Gender, age, and family size; infants or older people spend more than children or young adults; a family of five spends more than a single individual
Clinical characteristics	Heart disease, cancer, and diabetes; people with these diseases spend more than others either because of treatment of current problems or a higher propensity for future catastrophes, such as strokes
Socioeconomic factors	Income and education; poor individuals may have worse health in general and need more care; financial concerns may cause patients to present later in their illness when care will be more expensive
Cost-of-care factors	Living in an area where there are many hospital beds or where the wages of hospital workers are high may affect prices
Environmental factors	Exposure to toxic substances (e.g., radiation or lead) or hazardous conditions at home or work; workers in the mining and construction industry may need more health services than other workers

Table 9.2

Risk Adjusters and Their Sources

Risk Adjuster	Potential Data Source
Age	Enrollment, administrative, survey, clinical
Gender	Enrollment, administrative, survey, clinical
Family size	Enrollment, survey (not always captured)
Prior hospitalization	Administrative, clinical
Prior year's utilization	Administrative
Comorbid conditions	Clinical, administrative (limited)
Institutional status	Administrative
Welfare status	Survey, Medicaid, or Supplemental Security Income insurance enrollment files
County of residence	Enrollment, administrative, survey (may not be released for confidentiality reasons)
Health status	Survey
Functional status	Survey, Medicare (permanently disabled individuals), clinical

The highest-cost patients are generally not the most likely to die; therefore, adjusting payments requires the use of different risk adjusters or different weights from those used to adjust for differences in severity associated with health outcomes, such as death (discussed below). For example, those stroke patients who are likely to die within 30 days of being admitted to the hospital are not as expensive, on average, as less-sick patients who probably will not die but who will need months of physical therapy. However, in some cases the two methods overlap, and the adjusters may be the same between severity and risk-adjustment models. In the PPS/Quality of Care (QOC) study conducted by RAND (Keeler, 1991), many of the risk adjusters for hospital costs were also used to predict 30-day mortality. However, the relative importance (i.e., the weights) of these adjusters differed across the applications. Also, some factors were important only for predicting costs (e.g., whether the patient came from a nursing home) and were not predictive of patient outcomes (e.g., death). Nonetheless, many of the general rules for risk adjusting costs also apply to severity adjustment of health outcomes.

WHY IS RISK ADJUSTMENT IMPORTANT?

Risk adjustment is important now that many public and private purchasers pay on a *prospective* basis in an attempt to control spending on health care. Under PPS, medical care providers are reimbursed for the expected or average cost of caring for a patient, rather than the actual cost. Such payments create financial incentives to providers to deliver care more efficiently because spending in excess of expected payments reduces their profits.

Prospective payment systems of reimbursement were introduced by the federal government in 1984 for Medicare hospital admissions and, more recently, have been used in Medicaid managed care experiments. The annual capitation payments from insurers to medical groups, and within managed care organizations for selected benefits or "carveouts"—such as mental health and substance abuse services—also represent prospective payments. Prospective reimbursement has been successful in moderating the growth in health care costs (Russell and Manning, 1989; Luft and Morrison, 1991; Newhouse and the Insurance Experiment Group, 1993).

A health plan's or provider's costs will depend on at least four factors:

1. Patient characteristics (i.e., the types and numbers of cases or patients, often referred to as the case mix);

2. The efficiency of the provider;

3. The intensity of services or treatment provided; and,

4. Unpredictable events (e.g., chance or random factors, such as accidents).

The government and employers, who are the primary payors, are willing to compensate health plans and providers for higher costs related to differences in patient case mix. Payors also are generally willing to pay for higher quality care; although, recently, payors have been asking for evidence that health outcomes are really better at self-designated high-quality institutions. With large numbers of patients or enrollees, the costs associated with unpredictable events should average out, such that high costs related to a few accidents are offset by the low costs incurred by a large number of relatively healthy individuals. By contrast, payors are unwilling to pay for added costs that stem from inefficiency in the delivery of care.

Risk adjustment is one means for setting fair reimbursement rates for health plans (e.g., insurance premiums) and providers (e.g., capitation rates, usually in the form of a flat annual payment for each individual cared for) given different mixes of "health risks." If individuals randomly choose health plans, all insurers would enroll roughly equal shares of poor and good health risks. Some patients would be less expensive to care for than others, but on average, the cost of caring for patients would be covered. However, because of differences in the design of benefit packages and the ability of individuals to freely choose among plans, people who require or demand more health care services are likely to select more generous health plans.[1] Plans in which high users are concentrated will be at a cost disadvantage independent of how efficiently they provide care, if they are paid the average cost of the whole population.

There are two important reasons to account for differences in utilization and costs in setting reimbursement rates. First, if health plans and health care providers are underreimbursed when they care for a large number of sick (i.e., expensive) patients, they have a financial incentive to avoid enrolling these individuals. When insurers deliberately seek to provide coverage only to the healthiest individuals to minimize the costs they expect to incur, they are participating in a practice referred to as *risk selection*. Health plans attempt to select the best health risks by engaging in medical underwriting,[2] not offering products that would attract unhealthy enrollees, and requiring proof of insurability (i.e., prior coverage within the last three months). Risk selection can lead to large groups of individuals, many of whom may be in need of care (e.g., persons with AIDS or any preexisting condition), experiencing increased difficulty buying insurance. Risk adjustment can be used to ensure that providers are compensated appropriately for the number and types of patients they see (case mix) and thus reduce the incentive for risk selection.

Second, because it may be difficult to tell at enrollment who will be expensive, health plans and providers who are not adequately reimbursed for sicker people may reduce their costs by getting such people to disenroll. If health plans

---

[1]In the Federal Employees Health Benefits Plan (FEHBP), selection was estimated to raise the Blue Cross high-option premium 33 percent and to reduce the low-option premium 21 percent (Price and Mays, 1985).

[2]Medical underwriting is a process by which health insurance plans ask applicants about their health status, existing medical conditions, and prior utilization. The purpose is to identify unhealthy applicants and to either deny them coverage, exclude preexisting conditions from coverage, or charge them a higher premium so that the health plan does not lose money on them. Unfortunately, for people with high expected expenses, premiums may be set so high as to make purchasing coverage unattractive or unaffordable.

reduce the amount of care they provide for expensive patients, they can make themselves unattractive. This can be done either by limiting the care provided for a given condition or by limiting access to certain types of services that attract high users (e.g., limit the number of visits or amount of reimbursement for mental health and substance abuse care). Low quality for expensive patients may not be punished by the market, because without adequate reimbursement, no plan can afford to cover these patients. Plans may use this strategy as an alternative to risk selection.

Risk selection is not just a theoretical problem. HCFA currently pays Medicare HMOs a capitation rate (i.e., a fixed payment per person for all care received) that is 95 percent of the average fee-for-service rate of spending in the same county. One study found that Medicare beneficiaries spent only 77 percent of the average level for all fee-for-service beneficiaries in the year before they joined the HMO (Hill and Brown, 1990). By enrolling a healthier (i.e., less expensive in fee-for-service relative to the average) group of people, the HMOs could profit even without being more efficient in providing care. In another instance of risk selection, Blue Cross had to abandon community rating in the large-group insurance market after commercial insurers lured away healthier groups with lower premiums. For more on the evidence of risk selection and policy options to mitigate selection, see Newhouse (1994).

In summary, the purpose of risk adjustment is to adjust prospective payments to health plans or providers so as to avoid financially penalizing those that attract a sicker group of enrollees or patients. It is not designed to be used by health plans to select individuals. If each person's payment reflects what an average provider would spend on them, incentives to select favorable risks disappear. Furthermore, if payments were approximately equal to costs, health plans and providers could afford to specialize in treating particular groups of expensive patients (e.g., persons with AIDS or cancer).

HOW IS RISK ADJUSTMENT USED?

Risk adjustment is used to set health insurance premiums, to establish Medicare hospital payment rates, to determine capitated risk contracts, and to measure provider performance. The common thread is cost, because risk adjustment tries to account for differences in individuals that affect their use of health care services and the associated costs. In the examples that follow, the perspective of the person or group doing the adjusting may change, but the purpose of risk adjustment remains the same: to account for cost differences between groups of individuals.

Setting Private Health Insurance Premiums

Insurers currently use family size—which partly explains differences in health care utilization and costs—as a factor to adjust premiums. Premium prices may differ depending on whether the household contains a single person, a married couple without children, a single parent and child, or a family. Insurance premiums may also vary depending on the age of the worker. Adjustment at this level is crude because these two factors explain only a small portion of the observed variation in the use of services and costs. Still, these adjustment factors are often used because the information is easily obtained. Engaging in a more refined process of risk adjustment is challenging because information that may be important to predicting use and health care spending cannot be obtained or observed. Factors such as health status, preferences for health care, service use, and past health care spending may be predictive of future health care spending; yet these data are usually unavailable because of the lack of data, restrictions on gaining access to confidential data, or inability to measure the factor.

Purchasers could potentially use risk adjustment to level the playing field within the company with respect to how much they pay for each employee's coverage. Historically, employers have subsidized employees who have chosen more expensive forms of coverage (FFS plans) by making larger premium contributions for those employees than for employees who chose less-expensive managed care plans (HMOs, IPAs, and PPOs). This is now changing as illustrated by the University of California's decision to provide the same dollar contribution for each employee, regardless of the health plan chosen. The dollar amount was based on the cost of the least-expensive plan among the set of plan options. Employees who chose more expensive plans were required to pay the difference in the premium. As a result of this change in 1994, 25 percent of employees switched to cheaper plans that year. Virtually no employees shifted to more expensive plans (Buchmueller and Feldstein, 1995).

This system does not really level the playing field, however, because plans with a large number of inexpensive enrollees will have lower premiums for that reason alone. Therefore, employers should use risk adjustment of plan premiums to ensure that payments reflect the efficiency and intensity/quality of chosen plans and not the case mix of enrollees.

Establishing Hospital Payment Rates for Medicare

Medicare's PPS for hospital admissions, which is based on diagnosis related groups (DRGs), is another familiar risk-adjustment system. Instead of paying hospitals the same amount for each admission, DRGs use the patient's principal diagnosis and sometimes other factors (e.g., comorbid conditions) to define a payment that reflects the average cost of treating a person with that condition.

The method used to construct the DRG payment system is one that is frequently used to develop a risk-adjusted payment[3] and, at the broadest level of conceptualization, consists of the following steps:

- Group patients into clinical categories that are similar in terms of costs;

- Calculate the average cost for each group; and

- Use the average cost as the basis for payment for patients who fall within that group.

It is important to make sure that the reimbursement groups are homogeneous because if groups contain patients with widely differing costs, hospitals that treat more severely ill patients within the group will be underpaid. Since the inception of DRG payments, new DRGs have been added in response to the identification of DRG subgroups that differ sharply from the original DRG in their resource utilization. The identification of new DRG subgroups has led to payments that more accurately reflect the cost of caring for these patients. The current system contains 489 DRGs; however, HCFA has proposed a major revision that would further adjust for differences in risks and costs by accounting for the patient's secondary diagnosis (Edwards et al., 1994). Again, the purpose of the refinement is to more accurately predict the cost of caring for patients with given medical conditions so that providers are fairly reimbursed.

Determining Capitated Risk Contracts

Medicare has also developed a risk-adjustment system for setting capitated risk contracts for Medicare enrollees in HMOs and other capitated plans. The risk adjustment method is referred to as the Adjusted Average Per Capita Cost (AAPCC) system. The AAPCC system is used to set capitation rates for three groups of Medicare beneficiaries, who are eligible because of

- Age;

- Disabilities; or

- An end stage renal disease diagnosis.

The AAPCC uses age, gender, welfare status, institutional status, and county of residence to adjust for differences in costs. The AAPCC method of setting capitation rates is controversial. The method of adjustment has been widely criticized both for its limited predictive power (i.e., the method only explains 1

---

[3]A similar system, the Resource Utilization Group (RUG) system was developed using the same method. It is used to pay nursing home per diems in New York and several other states (Cornelius et al., 1994).

percent of the variation in individual costs) and the county adjustment factor, which gives higher rates to parts of the country that have uncontrolled Medicare spending.

The AAPCC risk-adjustment system and others illustrate that our present ability to predict prospectively much of the variation in health care spending is limited. Newhouse (1995) notes that only 20 to 25 percent of the variance in annual health care spending for a random sample of the population is predictable. To achieve this level requires including a person's self-assessed health status and the prior year's health care spending. Newhouse (1995), Swartz (1995) and others concede that achieving this level of predictive power requires a great deal of effort. Because no existing risk-adjustment system achieves high predictive power prospectively, some form of payment adjustment will still need to occur retrospectively. One illustration of this is the Medicare DRG system, which provides "outlier" payments to hospitals that have high-cost cases. The risk-adjustment model is inadequate for predicting the cost of treating these cases and HCFA provides a retrospective reimbursement to hospitals to compensate them for treating very expensive patients (this is described below).

Richard Kronick at the University of California, San Diego (UCSD), has been advising state Medicaid programs on how they might use risk adjustment prospectively to adjust Medicaid payments for patients with disabilities. By adjusting premium rates for patients with greater expected utilization of care, states help ensure high-quality care to low-income areas (Kronick et al., 1995). Currently, capitated health plans that receive a fixed payment based on the cost of treating the average patient are unwilling to make large investments in low-income areas or to develop innovative systems of care for persons with AIDS, end stage renal disease, and other chronic illnesses, because the prospect of incurring financial losses is large. Risk adjustment can be used to help ensure that appropriate payments are made to those insurers and providers who treat the poor and disabled. Kronick and colleagues (1995) have stated that for risk adjustment to work under these circumstances, regulation to reduce risk selection by health plans will be necessary. Kronick is attempting to group similar patients (i.e., those with disabilities) to predict resource use more accurately—an approach similar to the design of the DRG system. Work thus far has shown that costs are more predictable among the disabled—a more homogeneous group, given that conditions persist from year to year—but costs may vary greatly among patients with different disabilities (Kronick et al., 1995).

Profiling the Performance of Providers

Risk adjustment has also been used to ensure accurate *profiling* of the practice patterns and resource utilization of physicians, medical groups, and hospitals.

It is necessary to risk-adjust for differences in the patient populations treated by each of these groups to ensure a fair comparison. Examples of profiling study questions include: Do primary care physicians or specialists spend more resources on their patients? Do teaching hospitals have longer lengths of stay and higher costs than nonteaching hospitals? The validity of such studies depends greatly on how well they control for differences in the case mix of the patients treated. For example, if teaching hospitals treat the most difficult cases, you would expect their lengths of stay to be longer and their costs to be higher. However, if comparisons were made with similar types of patients (i.e., patients with the same medical problems) among institutions, the costs at teaching and nonteaching hospitals might or might not be different. Risk adjustment allows for a fair comparison to be made when the case mix is different.

In addition, private and public purchasers can use risk adjustment to evaluate provider cost. A self-insured company may have negotiated contracts with health plans that depend somewhat on how expensive the company's own enrollees would be for those providers to treat. This requires adjusting the data from the provider on current costs to standardize them to (or make them reflect) the people expected to enroll in the plan from the company. Contracts can then be negotiated at a price that is fair to both the purchaser and the provider.

Providers can also use risk adjustment in internal cost studies to assess efficiency. For example, in a study of the costs of obstetric care at eight Southern California Kaiser hospitals, the evaluation team controlled for case mix to determine which hospitals were more efficient. That is, they removed patient factors that influence the cost of treatment, independent of the care provided. The study found that staffing (i.e., the proportion of deliveries performed by midwives) and occupancy were more important than cesarean rates in determining case-mix-adjusted costs (Finkler and Wirtschaftler, 1991). The study also examined case-mix-adjusted birth outcomes, using a severity adjustment model, and found that outcomes were unrelated to costs. Controlling for differences in patients, by risk adjusting, allows providers to compare costs on an equal footing.

To see if better hospital quality saves money, researchers used risk adjustment to examine factors that influence hospital costs in a large sample of Medicare hospitalizations, making separate adjustments for costs and quality. They found that better quality hospitals were more expensive, even after adjusting for differences in teaching status, size, local wages, and whether they receive a disproportionate share of difficult cases. This held true even for measures of quality that might not be obviously expensive, such as better cognitive processes of nurses and doctors (Keeler et al., 1990).

HOW IS A RISK-ADJUSTMENT SYSTEM EVALUATED?

A risk-adjustment model or system can be relatively simple, including a few easy-to-obtain variables from administrative data (e.g., age, gender, and family size), or it might include many clinical variables (e.g., principal diagnosis, co-morbid conditions, and functional status) from medical records. Generally, the predictions will be more precise by including more variables in the model, but prediction variables may be omitted for reasons discussed below.

Predictions of future costs have been based on prior utilization, demographics, chronic diseases, and self-assessments of health or functional status. Newhouse (1986) identifies four criteria for evaluating a risk-adjustment system:

1. The strength with which the system predicts use and costs;

2. The size of incentives for inefficient care;

3. The ease of collecting the data; and

4. The ease of auditing and the difficulty of gaming the system.

A report by the White House Task Force on Health Risk Pooling (1993) contains a critical summary of current systems using similar evaluation criteria. Described below are examples of what each criterion assesses.

Strength of Predictions

All risk-adjustment systems face the problem that future health needs, and thus costs, are not very predictable. Major expenses, such as trauma or extreme prematurity at birth, are unexpected and inherently unpredictable. Even for people with chronic conditions (e.g., hypertension, diabetes, or asthma) who tend to use more care, the added expected expenses occur not primarily because of maintenance drug costs, but as a result of a higher chance of having a stroke or heart attack.

In particular, it is important to understand that most of the year-to-year differences in health spending among a group of individuals occur because of events, many of which are unexpected, that occur at the individual level (e.g., a new diagnosis of breast cancer or diabetes). Individual factors that do not change over time (e.g., gender, education, and race) do not help predict future costs (Newhouse et al., 1989, and 1993; van Vliet and van de Ven, 1992). As noted above, even if time-varying factors are included (e.g., health status or pregnancy status), at most about 20 percent of the total variation in health spending can be explained (Newhouse, 1995). However, explaining even small amounts of the difference in utilization can have important financial ramifications.

The limited ability of risk-adjustment systems to predict much of the variation in health spending is not a fatal flaw. If no one knows in advance which individuals within a group will be expensive, and the payments for the group as a whole are correct, then risk adjustment works. Providers can benefit from risk selection only to the extent that they can predict better than the risk-adjustment formula. The AAPCC explains only 1 percent of the variation in spending, whereas newer systems such as the Diagnostic Cost Groups (DCGs) and Ambulatory Cost Groups (ACGs) that incorporate health measures based on prior utilization may explain more than 5 percent of the variation in spending. This represents a significant improvement in a rate setter's ability to predict spending. However, because expenses are concentrated among a small group in the population (i.e., the top 5 percent spend 58 percent of all health care dollars, see Berk and Monheit, 1992), the profits can be large if additional information above that used by the rate setter allows a plan to keep out just a few expensive people (Newhouse et al., 1989). If people remained enrolled in health plans for longer periods of time, instead of shifting fairly frequently, the concentration of expenses and therefore selection would not be as important. Roos et al., (1989) showed that among the Manitoba elderly, cumulative spending over many years was much less concentrated than during a shorter time period. Expenses were spread, in part, because death, which is associated with very high costs in the six months before the event, occurs only once per person.

Incentives for Inefficient Care

Adjusting premiums based on prior utilization has an additional problem in that it may reward health plans that provide inefficient care. For example, prior hospitalizations are a big cost factor, and HMOs that have been able to reduce hospital admissions argue that providing additional premium payments for prior hospitalizations penalizes them (i.e., they will have fewer hospitalizations and therefore will receive lower payments). Unfortunately, prior utilization is the factor that explains the largest portion of explainable variation in costs between people (e.g., if 20 percent of the variation can be explained, 10 percent of that would be attributable to prior utilization).

Ease of Collecting Data

Again, the data required to conduct risk adjustment may not be found in a single data source and primary data collection may be needed. As discussed below (see the subsection entitled What Data Sources Are Available for Severity

Adjustment?) and in Chapter Five, the utility of a risk adjuster to the risk-adjustment system is related to its ability to predict future costs relative to the feasibility and cost of obtaining data on the risk adjuster. A few risk adjusters, such as age, are available from enrollment files, administrative data, and medical records and therefore are frequently used. Other adjusters, such as health status, are less frequently used because they require a special survey.

Ease of Audit and Gaming the System

Risk adjustment can lead to changes in the data on which payments are based. A review of the average DRG weights for Medicare hospital admissions shows that the severity of cases (e.g., the case mix) has risen over time. Under the DRG payment system, as case mix rises, so do payments to hospitals. Some of the increase in case mix is due to general trends toward the increased use of expensive surgical procedures, especially cardiac surgery, in the elderly population. However, a portion of the increase has occurred because of differences in the coding of cases after the introduction of the DRG system, which was a result of hospitals' efforts to receive the maximum payment for a case. The coding changes are referred to as "DRG creep" and have been well-studied (Carter et al., 1990). Some of the creep is due to hospitals' coding diagnoses that were always present but not always coded previously (e.g., ventilator use), because at that time hospitals received payment for all services rendered, independent of the patient's diagnosis code. DRG creep also occurs because hospitals use software to identify which diagnoses for a patient will obtain the maximum DRG payment. The key point is that when data are used to decide how much a provider is reimbursed, the data reported will be affected by the desire for higher payments.

WHAT CAN BE DONE TO AUGMENT PROSPECTIVE RISK ADJUSTMENT?

Because of the limited ability to predict costs prospectively, it has been advocated that prospective payments be supplemented with retrospective payments to prevent risk selection and undertreatment. This strategy is used in the Medicare PPS. Retrospective adjustments to payments is another way to ensure that providers are fairly compensated for all types of patients they treat. However, financing a retrospective payment generally involves reducing the initial prospective amount paid.

Three common methods are used to reimburse retrospectively:

- **First dollar reinsurance** simply pays a fraction of the total costs. It is a type of insurance that insurers or self-funded plans buy to protect themselves against specified, rare, and high-priced risks, such as heart transplantation. Reinsurance further spreads the financial risk. For example, with 25 percent reinsurance, the central payor pays $2,500 to the hospital for a stay costing $10,000.

- **Individual outlier payments** are characterized by a loss threshold and an insurance rate. For example, when costs exceed the threshold, the provider gets the outlier insurance rate multiplied by the actual costs incurred beyond the threshold. Therefore, if the outlier insurance rate is 20 percent, and the actual costs beyond the threshold are $2,000, the outlier payment would be $400.

- **Event payments** are allotments for expensive episodes of illness, such as end stage renal disease or bone marrow transplants. Such events must be clearly defined and occur in a manner that is unaffected by the payment. The amount of the payment is a high fraction of the cost that would be incurred by an average provider. Event payments differ from outlier payments in that they are independent of actual costs incurred by the provider.

Giving providers any relief from bearing the costs of treatment may lead to wasteful overuse. However, in a competitive and informed market, the waste from increased spending caused by limited and targeted retrospective payments will be small. At present, hospitals bear little of the costs of the hospital care of those insured with a FFS health plan, whereas capitated HMOs and other managed care plans bear all or a significant portion of these costs. The different financial incentives lead to a large variation in the use of hospital care between FFS and capitated health plans. Generally, a low uniform level of reinsurance would reduce overall incentives for excess hospital care and also reduce variation in hospital use (Ellis and McGuire, 1993).

WHAT WORK IS BEING DONE TO IMPROVE THE ABILITY TO RISK-ADJUST?

The use of prospective payment to control the growth in health care spending and the recent health care reform debate have generated interest in better adjustment of premiums to account for differences in patient risks. In response, HCFA has funded work to improve methods to predict utilization and expenditures. Two approaches currently being tested are described below.

Predicting Costs Based on Prior Hospitalization

Ash et al. (1989), at Boston University, have developed a system to predict costs that is based on information about prior hospitalizations. The system, DCGs, specifically ignores discretionary hospitalizations and some one- or two-day hospitalizations. This reflects a decision not to reward providers for hospitalizing patients who could have been treated as outpatients. It also serves to make the system more difficult for hospitals to manipulate ("game") to secure a higher payment in the following year. The method used by Ash and her colleagues required grouping 104 clinically coherent hospital diagnostic groups into nine similar cost groups. The largest group was "no hospitalizations in the prior year," and the other groups consisted of "hospitalization of type X in the prior year." To minimize the number of groups, Ash et al. used the "worst" hospitalization of the prior year to classify individuals. The dependent variable was dollars per month spent by individuals. This model explains about 5 percent of the observed variation in Medicare expenditures.

Predicting Outpatient Care Costs

Another risk-adjustment method under development attempts to predict only the ambulatory care portion of costs for the next year. The method defines ACGs, and uses age, gender, and ICD-9 visit diagnosis codes in year 1 as risk adjusters to predict ambulatory costs in year 2. The initial system explained 50 percent of the variation in ambulatory costs retrospectively and 20 percent prospectively, using 51 ACG categories.[4] It is interesting to note that as research continues to improve these systems, the DCGs and ACGs are converging—that is, DCGs have added data from ambulatory care diagnoses and ACGs have added information about prior hospitalizations to predict variation in resource utilization.

WHAT IS SEVERITY ADJUSTMENT?

The purpose of severity adjustment (sometimes referred to as severity-of-illness adjustment) is to allow for a "fair" comparison of health outcomes, such as death or disability level. Comparing health outcomes is one way to evaluate the quality of care. A number of health outcomes can be measured and compared. A few of these are defined in Table 9.3.

Although we might like to compare mortality rates or functional status after a particular type of surgery, it is important to recognize that patients who die or recover more slowly after an operation may not have received poorer quality

---

[4]The distribution of ambulatory spending is less skewed and more predictable than inpatient spending, which accounts for the higher level of explanatory power (Weiner et al., 1991; Newhouse et al., 1989 and 1993). Although spending for ambulatory care is a substantial part of total spending on health care, the costs represent only a small part of the variation in overall year-to-year spending.

Table 9.3

Selected Health Care Outcomes, Their Definitions, and Examples

Outcome	Definition	Example
Mortality	Death within a specified time frame from a condition or following an intervention such as surgery	The 30-day mortality rate for patients hospitalized with acute myocardial infarction was 24.2 percent (735 patients out of a total of 3,037 died within 30 days) (Blumberg, 1991)
Morbidity	The health problems (e.g., pain) or complications (e.g., infection) that occur as a result of a condition or its treatment	Morbidity related to CABG surgery includes the need for prolonged ventilator support after surgery (Higgins et al., 1992); morbidity related to hip or knee replacement surgery includes the inability to walk without assistance
Health-related quality of life	A multidimensional concept that describes a person's overall well-being as it relates to health problems and their treatment; dimensions describe physical functioning as well as emotional and social well-being	Ratings are often on a 0–100 scale, with 0 representing poor quality of life and 100 representing excellent quality of life; patients are usually asked to rate their own quality of life over a specified time period (e.g., past week or past month)

care but may have been sicker before treatment. Patient characteristics such as age, severity of illness (e.g., localized cancer vs. cancer that has spread throughout the body), and comorbidities or secondary conditions (e.g., the patient experiencing an acute myocardial infarction is also diabetic) place patients at different risks for outcomes before receiving care. Severity adjustment is used to refer to adjustments made both to reflect the severity of the disease that is the focus of treatment (e.g., heart disease for bypass surgery) and the overall illness level of the patient, including comorbid conditions (e.g., diabetes). Because both types of severity can contribute to the likelihood of achieving good outcomes, both are included in severity-adjustment models. By accounting for these baseline patient characteristics or risk factors, severity adjustment enables valid comparisons of health outcomes to be made by "leveling the playing field" (Iezzoni et al., 1994).

WHY IS SEVERITY ADJUSTMENT IMPORTANT?

In the absence of severity adjustment, comparisons of health outcomes are made that are often false and may lead to incorrect conclusions and actions. For example, hospital mortality data were some of the first outcome statistics widely publicized that demonstrated the importance of severity adjustment. In 1986, HCFA released hospital-level mortality figures without adequately adjusting for the types of patients seen at each hospital (i.e., case mix) (Berwick and Wald, 1990). HCFA reported that 142 hospitals had significantly higher death rates than predicted, whereas 127 had significantly lower rates. The institution with the highest death rate (87.6 percent of Medicare patients died compared to a predicted rate of 22.5 percent) was a hospice caring for terminally ill patients. In this case, the high mortality rate was not a reflection of poor-quality care but of the preferences of an acutely ill patient population with a very high risk of death.

Patients with the same principal diagnosis or primary condition but different comorbidities may face varying risks of death. Comorbidities or other conditions that patients may have in addition to their principal diagnosis can have a dramatic effect on patient outcomes. For example, a study of 2,935 cancer patients treated in seven California hospitals found that the three hospitals with mortality rates significantly greater than the statewide average were also identified as having the highest comorbidity (Greenfield et al., 1988). Again, without adequately adjusting for differences in severity of illness, hospitals were incorrectly identified as having higher-than-average mortality rates.

Without severity adjustment, information may be inaccurate, misleading, or simply wrong. Furthermore, incentives will exist for health plans and medical groups to select the healthiest enrollees to improve performance (e.g., to demonstrate that they have lower mortality and morbidity). More and more, information about health outcomes serves as the basis for policy decisions by providers, insurers, and employers. If there is an interest in comparing health outcomes, severity adjustment will be necessary.

HOW IS SEVERITY ADJUSTMENT USED?

This section is devoted to understanding when and how to use severity adjustment. The following questions will be addressed with an illustration of how to approach each point:

- When is severity adjustment necessary?
- What risk factors should be considered for adjustment?
- What data sources are available?

When Is Severity Adjustment Necessary?

Generally, severity adjustment is needed when

- External factors influence the results;
- The external factors are nonrandomly distributed in the groups being compared; and

- The relationship between these factors and the result of interest is understood.

External factors pertain to such things as patient age, gender, presence of other illnesses (i.e., comorbidities), and acuity (i.e., urgency of treatment). An example of a nonrandom distribution is a situation where one hospital in a city receives the majority of urgent coronary bypass patients because it specializes in treating these types of cases, whereas other hospitals treat primarily elective cases. With respect to bypass surgery, the relationship between urgency of the operation and mortality is well-understood (i.e., urgent cases have worse mortality outcomes than elective cases).

Several steps, as illustrated below, can help an analyst evaluate whether severity adjustment is required.

Step 1: Define the specific question you wish to answer. How the question is defined will influence the analytic approach taken (see also Chapter Six).

The question should address the following issues:

- What is the condition (e.g., breast cancer or management of adult asthma) or procedure (e.g., CABG surgery) of interest?

- What is the time frame for evaluation? This may be affected by the condition or procedure of interest as well as data concerns. Longer time frames increase the likelihood that external factors will influence outcomes.

- What is/are the outcome(s) of interest? The outcome should be related to the treatment or condition and should be measurable.

- What is the purpose of the study? Think of the audience (e.g., providers, employers, or patients) and the ultimate purpose of this information (e.g., internal quality assurance or provide employers with comparative data on health plans).

Example questions include:

1. What is the 30-day mortality rate for patients receiving CABG surgery in hospital A between 1992 and 1997?

2. What percentage of women between ages 50 and 74 covered by health plan A received a mammogram in 1997?

3. How does the emergency department admission rate for adult asthma patients covered by health plan A compare to the rate for adult asthma patients covered by health plan B?

A complete definition of the study question or condition helps to ensure that the outcome being assessed is constructed properly. For example, the time frame in question 1 is relevant because a longer postoperative period may include mortality from causes unrelated to CABG. In question 2, there is no consensus that women under age 50 or over age 74 should be receiving annual mammograms and therefore women outside the age range 50–74 may be included in the study population. In question 3, care is focused on emergency department visits only, so that any identified differences can potentially be tracked back to problems with outpatient management, a central component of asthma management.

Step 2: Once a study question is defined, determine whether severity adjustment is needed and, if so, possible.

Assess whether patient characteristics or other factors are likely to have a large effect on the outcome. These factors might involve

- The clinical reason patients had the procedure or principal diagnosis;

- The severity of the disease;

- The presence of comorbid conditions; and

- Other factors (e.g., sociodemographics or attitudes about health care).

Applying this process to the example questions in Step 1:

1. What is the 30-day mortality rate for patients receiving CABG surgery in hospital A between 1992 and 1997?

In this question, a procedure rather than an illness is specified. CABG surgery is indicated for several principal diagnoses, such as unstable angina and congestive heart failure, which may have different probabilities of mortality following surgery. Attention should be focused on how to identify the clinical reason for which patients received CABG surgery so that the case mix can be accounted for in estimating mortality. Also, you may wish to exclude those who had multiple surgical procedures (e.g., valve replacement with CABG surgery).

The severity of the disease will vary, making some patients more susceptible to complications and death after CABG surgery. Since these characteristics cannot be made equal across all patients, it is crucial to account for pretreatment differences in patients through severity adjustment. These pretreatment characteristics include clinical factors such as the degree of cardiac dysfunction (e.g., the number of vessels involved and the degree of stenosis), urgency of the operation, and the preoperative hematocrit (Higgins et al., 1992).

The number and severity of comorbid or coexisting conditions will vary, making some patients more susceptible to complications and death after CABG surgery. Important comorbidities include diabetes mellitus and cerebrovascular disease.

Other surgical risk factors (e.g., patient age) may affect outcomes.

The basic purpose in this step is to make the group as homogeneous as possible with respect to the outcome (mortality), either by excluding persons who are likely to have different outcomes or by adjusting for factors that contribute to differential outcomes.

2. What percentage of women between ages 50 and 74 covered by health plan A received a screening mammogram in 1997?

In general, all women between the ages of 50 and 74 should receive an annual mammogram to improve the likelihood of identifying cancer at an early stage, except those who have had or are currently under treatment for breast cancer. By excluding persons who are clinically different, it is not necessary to further categorize patients by principal diagnosis, severity of principal diagnosis, or comorbidity, since these factors will not influence the result—whether the woman received an annual mammogram. Severity adjustment may not be necessary in this case.

However, it might be interesting for improvement purposes to discover where lower rates are concentrated: by zip code, age group, or benefits package.

3. How does the emergency department admission rate for adult asthma patients covered by health plan A compare to the rate for adult asthma patients covered by health plan B?

High emergency department (ED) utilization rates are often used as a proxy for inadequate ambulatory care. In this question, all patients have the same principal diagnosis, but comorbidities and the severity of each patients' asthma condition may differ.

The severity of a patient's asthma may affect the patient's likelihood of seeking care in the ED. Adjustment for the severity of the principal diagnosis is necessary, because if one health plan has a higher proportion of patients with asthma who are severely ill, it may also have a higher ED admission rate than another health plan, even if quality of care in the two plans is the same.

The number and severity of comorbid conditions will vary among patients. For example, some patients may have coexisting heart disease, which can make an asthma exacerbation more life-threatening and make those patients more likely to enter the ED.

Environmental factors (e.g., dust, presence of pets, or exposure to air pollution) in a patient's home or workplace can affect the probability of exacerbations and in turn the likelihood of seeking care in the ED. Health plans may have differing numbers of people who are exposed to these environmental triggers and may not be able to affect the likelihood of certain exposures.

These examples demonstrate that there are varying ways to identify which questions require severity adjustment. Most, if not all, outcome measures and many process of care measures will need to be adjusted for differences in population risk. Regardless of the study question, it is important to proceed through the above steps to be able to determine whether there is a need for severity adjustment. Severity adjustment is a complicated process and a clear presentation of the study question and its goals will help ensure the development of a parsimonious model.

What Factors Should Be Considered for Adjustment?

Once you decide you need to adjust for differences in severity, how do you choose the risk factors to include in a *severity-adjustment model* or *system*? The key is to focus on those factors (e.g., patient age) known to affect the result (e.g., death) and that are not likely to be modifiable by the entity being assessed (e.g., hospital or physician). Selecting risk factors and developing a severity-adjustment system involve taking a closer look at why you decided to adjust for severity in the first place. The categories previously identified—principal diagnosis, severity of illness, and comorbidities—are three of the most common dimensions of risk you might include in a severity measure. Depending on how narrow the question is, the principal diagnosis and certain severity criteria or comorbidities may also serve as inclusion or exclusion criteria for the study. For example, in question 3, the study population is restricted to adult patients with a principal diagnosis of asthma. A number of other dimensions of risk could be measured, including age, gender, acute clinical stability (current physiologic status of patient), and patient preferences. The various dimensions of risk that might need adjustment are shown in Table 9.4.

These dimensions contain several possible factors that could be incorporated into the development of a severity-adjustment system. Deciding which factors should be adjusted will require balancing the costs and benefits of including each factor in a severity-adjustment system designed to answer the study question. For example, how difficult is it to obtain data on the risk factor? If the risk factor is not included in the model, will the results still be meaningful and valid?

Table 9.4

Dimensions of Risk, Their Definitions, and Examples

Dimension	Definition	Examples
Age	Patient age, years	Given comparable clinical situations, most older patients are at higher risk for worse outcomes than younger patients
Gender	Male or female	Women metabolize some antihypertensive drugs more slowly then men; in general, women have a longer life expectancy than men
Acute clinical stability	The current physiologic status of the patient in terms of basic measures of bodily function	Vital signs, blood counts, and level of consciousness are examples; these factors identify whether the patient is at imminent risk of death
Principal diagnosis	The leading or primary disease that brings the patient into contact with the health care system	A patient with diabetes who enters the emergency room with chest pain will receive a principal diagnosis of acute myocardial infarction; diabetes is a comorbidity
Severity of principal diagnosis	The extent and nature of the patient's principal diagnosis based on expectations about the patient's clinical outcomes (e.g., death, functional status)	A patient whose prostate cancer is localized to the gland has a better prognosis (e.g., length of survival) than a patient whose prostate cancer has spread to the bone
Extent and severity of comorbidities	The number and severity of co-existing diagnoses separate from the principal diagnosis	Patients entering the ED with an acute myocardial infarction may also be diabetic and have rheumatoid arthritis; in addition, the patient's diabetes may be insulin- or noninsulin-dependent; the diabetes may affect the patient's chance of survival and the arthritis might affect return to normal function
Physical functional status	The ability to perform basic activities of daily living (e.g., feeding, bathing, dressing, shopping, cooking, using transportation)	A variety of measures are available for use by providers or patients to assess patient physical functional status; physical functional status may be an important risk factor that predicts outcomes (e.g., functional level before hip fracture may predict level of functioning posttreatment) as well as an outcome itself
Psychological, cognitive, and psychosocial functioning	The ability to appreciate and interact with other individuals, the capacity to understand information about one's health, and the presence of a social support network	A study that followed patients after acute myocardial infarction found that having a spouse or confidant reduced the risk of cardiac death (Williams et al., 1992)

Table 9.4 (continued)

Dimension	Definition	Examples
Cultural, ethnic, and socioeconomic attributes and behaviors	Attributes, beliefs, and behaviors derived from cultural, ethnic, and socioeconomic traits	Low socioeconomic status has been associated with higher mortality, possibly due to delays in access to care or chronic deprivations (e.g., malnutrition)
Health status and health-related quality of life	This category encompasses severity of illness, physical, psychosocial, and emotional functioning and well-being, and overall health-related quality of life	A variety of measures are available for use by patients and surrogates (e.g., providers or family members) to assess health status and quality of life; health status and health-related quality of life may predict outcomes as well as being outcomes themselves
Patient attitudes and preferences for outcomes	Patient's philosophy toward treatment that is based on beliefs, goals, and understanding of prognosis and therapeutic options	Depending on the decrease in the risk of recurrence and treatment toxicity, some breast cancer patients may choose chemotherapy and others may not

SOURCE: Adapted from Iezzoni (1997).

The following list of four questions should be asked when identifying factors for inclusion in a severity-adjustment system.

1. **Has severity adjustment previously been used in a well-regarded study of the condition, procedure, or outcome?** In all likelihood, your problem is one that someone else has studied. Not only may this prior work help you decide which risk factors are important to include in your severity-adjustment system, you may also find that a suitable measure already exists. Examples of existing systems and guidelines for evaluating them are described in the section below entitled How to Choose a Severity-Adjustment System.

2. **How does the clinical literature classify the disease of interest?** For example, most cancers are classified according to disease stage, clinical test results, and symptom status. Angina is classified according to criteria from the New York State Cardiac Society. Consensus about severity classification is one signal that this factor may be important to account for in interpreting results.

3. **Do the identified pretreatment characteristics affect the risk for the outcome of interest?** For example, the five-year survival rate (outcome) for patients with localized breast cancer is significantly greater than for patients whose cancer has spread to their lungs and bone. Patients with decreased cardiac function undergoing CABG surgery are at greater risk for death than patients with preserved function.

4. **How does the information provided by the risk factor compare to the ease or difficulty of obtaining accurate information about the risk factor?** For example, some clinical information can be found in encounter data, but the detail necessary for many study questions will probably require medical chart review by trained personnel, which is costly and time-consuming. In addition, some risk factors, such as cultural, ethnic, and socioeconomic attributes and behaviors, may require a special survey. You will need to decide whether adjusting for each particular factor is important enough (i.e., if it affects the outcome sufficiently) to justify the costs of data collection. Tradeoffs will have to be made between the importance of obtaining information and its cost. Consultation with clinicians and statisticians will probably be necessary to fully understand the tradeoffs. The advantages and disadvantages of using different data sources are explained in the next subsection.

Identifying the most important risk factors for inclusion in a severity-adjustment system or model requires effort, but without this effort, the information ultimately generated may be no more meaningful than it was without severity adjustment may be misleading.

What Data Sources Are Available for Severity Adjustment?

The choice of the data source affects the reliability (consistency with which results are produced) and validity (accuracy with which concept is measured) of the severity-adjustment system. Three currently available data sources contain information useful for severity adjustment. These data sources are defined below and are described in more detail in Chapter Five .

- **Administrative data** are generated from an interaction between a patient and provider (either ambulatory or inpatient) and they mainly contain information about the costs and services provided. Much of the information describing a hospital visit comes in the form of a *discharge abstract.*

- **Clinical data** can be found in the medical record, computerized laboratory results, and pharmacy records. Blood pressure, white blood count, and medications prescribed are examples of data that can be obtained from this source.

- **Survey data** are collected from routine or special surveys of individuals, especially patients. Surveys are used to assess patient satisfaction, preferences, and health-related quality of life (e.g., functional status).

Each potential data source has advantages and disadvantages for severity adjustment. It is important to understand the advantages and disadvantages of each data source for the purpose of severity adjustment. The characteristics of each also must be weighed relative to the goals of the study and available resources. For example, patient survey data are necessary for a study of the quality of life of patients one year after CABG surgery, but they are probably not necessary for an evaluation of the 30-day mortality rate following CABG surgery.

An example study question and a discussion of how cost and the severity-adjustment process are affected by the data source are described below.

1. Study Question

What is the change in functional status of patients age 50 or older one year after total hip replacement surgery received in 1997?

- **What is the condition or procedure?** *Hip replacement.* There is more than one indication for hip surgery, but arthritis is a significant cause. Therefore, this study question will be limited to total hip replacement surgery resulting from arthritis among those age 50 and older.

- **What is the specific time frame?** *One year* (in this case functional status is assessed one year after surgery in calendar year 1997). This allows patients enough time to reach full recovery. Evaluations conducted using shorter time periods may describe outcomes that reflect acute symptoms after surgery.

- **What is the outcome?** *Change in functional status.* This is the outcome of interest that might be defined or operationalized as physical functioning (e.g., ability to walk up and down stairs), role functioning (e.g., ability to complete household tasks), and number of disability days. Baseline measures of functional status should be obtained before surgery. Outcome measures should be obtained one year after surgery (this, of course, requires prospective evaluation).

In our example, the study question is well-defined because it is sufficiently specific and has an acceptable rationale for each choice.

2. Determine Whether Severity Adjustment Is Needed

- **Does severity of the principal diagnosis affect outcomes?** Yes. Arthritis severity will vary among patients. One way to measure severity is to determine whether patients had previous joint surgery. Another way is to administer a survey to the patients before surgery that asks about pain and limitations in physical functioning.

- **Does the outcome vary by comorbidity status?** Yes. Other secondary conditions (e.g., coronary artery disease or asthma) may also limit functional status and affect the rate and degree of recovery.

- **Does the outcome vary by any other patient characteristics?** Yes. Age, gender, education, and marital status, in addition to clinical factors such as preoperative comorbidities, have been shown to be significant predictors of functional status at one year (Greenfield et al., 1993).

This is a clear case in which severity adjustment is necessary; the next step is to identify risk factors and potential data sources if a suitable severity-adjustment system is not available.

3. Evaluate Data Sources

The following is a summary of the information that can be obtained from each data source (administrative, clinical, and survey) as well as the expected cost of abstracting the data.

- Administrative data

  — Cost per record: minimal, since most information will be available on-line; a programmer paid $10 to $15 per hour might extract data for analysis from the larger system within a few days.

  — Clinical data: type of fracture, comorbidities.

  — Patient-derived data: none.

  — Other data: demographic information such as age and gender; resource utilization data (e.g., length of stay and charges).

Summary: Severity adjustment is largely limited to information provided by ICD-9-CM codes and, as noted in Chapter Seven, it may be difficult to distinguish complications of care from comorbidities. The outcome of interest, functional status, is not documented.

- Clinical data (medical record)

  — Cost per record: $100/record (chart abstraction by trained personnel, including data checks) for a 45-minute abstraction form; need to factor in time to locate chart(s) (there may be several), abstract data, refile chart, keypunch data.

  — Clinical data: type of fracture, details of comorbidities, functional assessment reported by provider.

— Patient-derived data: only information reported to clinician that was subsequently documented (e.g., location and extent of pain).

— Other data: demographic information such as age and gender; length of stay, utilization of services (e.g., physical therapy); race/ethnicity may be available in some charts.

Summary: Data are good for severity adjustment because they include the principal diagnosis, comorbidities, and possibly pre- and postsurgery functional status. Functional status after one year will probably not be consistently documented. Some brief assessment may be available if ambulatory records are linked to inpatient records. Documentation may also be more likely for patients experiencing problems (poor outcomes) than for those doing well, so the data from this source may be biased.

- Survey data

— Cost per record: varies ($5–$20 per completed survey), depending on size of sample and mode of administration, and efforts to achieve high response rates.

— Clinical data: information on patient-reported comorbidities, symptoms, and functional status.

— Patient-derived data: information can be extensive depending on the type of measures (e.g., generic health status measures such as the RAND Short-Form 36) and items (e.g., How many disability days did you take over the past month?) chosen to assess functional status and the length of the survey.

— Resource utilization data: limited and based on patient self-report (recall over a one-year period may be unreliable).

Summary: Severity adjustment is limited to patient-reported comorbidities and the reliability of this information is questionable. However, the outcome of interest, functional status, can be comprehensively measured.

As this comparison demonstrates, more than one data source may be necessary to obtain all of the information needed to answer a study question. Alternatively, the question may be revised so that one data source is sufficient. Table 9.5 provides a comparison of the general advantages and disadvantages of each data source.

Finally, if an existing severity-adjustment system is used, the data source will be specified by the system. Therefore, if a severity-adjustment system is used rather than developed "from scratch," it is important to evaluate the system,

Table 9.5

A Comparison of Four Data Sources for Severity Adjustment

		Information Provided for:	
Data Source	Cost	Clinical Factors	Patient-Assessed Factors
Administrative	Low	Limited	None
Clinical (medical record)	Moderate to high[a]	Extensive	Limited to provider documentation of patient reports
Survey	Moderate	Limited to patient self-report	Extensive

[a]Depending on extent of automation.

including what data source it depends on. The data source as well as the risk factors included in a severity-adjustment system can lead to different results and the reader is encouraged to review articles that compare severity-adjustment systems and data sources (Iezzoni, 1992; Iezzoni, 1997; Romano, 1993; Daley, 1994; Kahn et al., 1992; and Hadorn et al., 1993).

HOW TO CHOOSE A SEVERITY-ADJUSTMENT SYSTEM

If severity adjustment is necessary to answer the question of interest, and one or more severity-adjustment systems exist for potential use, the next step is to evaluate each system. This is a difficult process and you may want to consult experts such as statisticians and the authors of a particular system. If one or more potentially suitable severity-adjustment systems are available for use, it is worth taking the time to summarize the major components of each system. At this point, some systems may be eliminated because they are not appropriate for your study question. For example, the outcomes being measured by many systems will not be the outcome you are interested in. In addition, if the goal is to compare health outcomes to assess quality of care, it is important to address whether there is a relationship between the outcome (e.g., 30-day mortality or ability to walk) and the condition (e.g., acute myocardial infarction) or procedure (e.g., hip fracture surgery) of interest. The final step is to try to assess the performance of the system. If severity adjustment is inadequate, the results can be misleading or simply wrong. If this is the case, building a severity-adjustment system from scratch may be necessary but should not be undertaken before exhausting all other options.

The first distinction to be made is whether the condition in question is a hospital or ambulatory condition. Most work to date has focused on hospital conditions. Second, this section has focused on *severity adjustment of health outcomes*. As previously mentioned, many systems have been created for risk adjustment of *costs* (e.g., resource utilization, costs, and charges). The systems are not substitutes for one another, so you need to make sure that you have one designed for the right purpose. Although some systems that focus on costs (discussed in the first half of this chapter) have subsequently been modified for studies of health outcomes with moderate success (Iezzoni, 1997), you should be cautious about using systems designed for one purpose in a context that is different from the original intent.

The following section provides a framework to identify the major components of a severity-adjustment system. Specifically, two hospital-based severity–adjustment systems and two ambulatory-based systems are presented. Each system is concerned with different outcomes, but each outcome can be used as a screen for quality of care. Although health outcomes are interesting in and of themselves, one driving issue behind severity adjustment of health outcomes is to be able to compare quality of care among health care delivery systems. As previously mentioned, this is an extremely important principle to keep in mind when each system is reviewed. The two hospital systems are (1) MedisGroups (original version), a generic system (not based on a principal diagnosis), and (2) the Computerized Severity Index (CSI), a diagnosis-specific system. Both systems have been studied extensively and continually undergo revision (Iezzoni, 1989; Blumberg, 1991; Iezzoni and Moskowitz, 1988; Iezzoni and Daley, 1992; Iezzoni, 1997). The methodology is less well developed on the ambulatory care side, but in this section two new systems are evaluated and compared: (1) an asthma severity-adjustment system currently being developed at Johns Hopkins University as part of the Managed Health Care Association Outcomes Management System Project (Steinwachs et al., 1995), and (2) a severity-adjustment system based on 15 different diseases treated in ambulatory settings that was developed as part of the Type II Diabetes Patient Outcomes Research Team project (Greenfield et al., 1995).

The following review of these severity-adjustment systems focuses on the key components of each system, including:

- **Outcome(s) and study population:** This includes the health outcomes the system was designed to assess and how the outcome is defined or operationalized. In addition, the population on which the system was tested should be identified.

- **Severity measure:** This component includes the definition of severity, risk factors included, and the framework used to assess severity for subsequent adjustment.

- **Disease-specific vs. generic system:** Most systems are *disease specific*, that is, severity is not defined independent of the principal diagnosis. This is because disease-specific systems are better able to predict outcomes than generic systems. Because such a large number of diseases exist, diagnoses are usually grouped into categories according to the organ system affected or some other scheme. Some systems are *generic* or defined independent of diagnosis. Generic systems typically perform poorly when contrasted with disease-specific systems.

- **Scoring system:** This includes the actual scale used to assign a severity score, the timing of scores, and the resources needed; in particular are specific software programs and computer expertise required?

- **Data source requirements:** This includes the actual data source (e.g., survey, clinical, or administrative) as well as the personnel needed to obtain and manage the data (e.g., medical record abstractors who may or may not be clinicians, data managers, or research assistants).

MedisGroups (Original Version)

MedisGroups is a severity-adjustment system that has been mandated for use in Pennsylvania since 1986 for its statewide cardiac procedures reporting system; more recently it has been used in Iowa and Colorado (Iezzoni et al., 1991). The corporate headquarters of MedisGroups is MediQual Systems, Inc., in Westborough, Massachusetts. All purchasers of the MedisGroups severity-scoring system contribute information to the MedisGroups Comparative Database, which represents about 450 hospitals (Iezzoni et al., 1993). The key components of the *original* MedisGroups system include:

- **Outcome(s):** The outcome measured is in-hospital mortality and the relevant patient population is all hospitalized patients.

- **Severity measure:** Severity is defined as the "risk of imminent organ failure." Severity is measured by using a scoring process (described below) that weights each abnormal finding out of a possible 550 (original number). Abnormal findings include such items as bowel inflammation on colonoscopy, hematocrit of less than 0.20, and an arterial pH of less than 7.15.

- **Generic:** Diagnosis is not used for adjustment, because it was believed that the risk of imminent organ failure would be comparable for all patients.

- **Scoring system:** Scores range from 0 ("no significant findings" or low severity) to 4 ("critical findings indicating the presence of organ failure" or high severity) at admission to the hospital, and a midstay review produces an assessment of morbidity (no morbidity, morbid, or major morbidity). Admission review includes the first 48 hours after admission and the midstay review generally encompasses days 5 through 7. In the original version, clinical judgment was used to develop final scores, which would require the expertise not only of clinicians but also of statisticians and possibly computer programmers. The revised version uses computer modeling, specifically logistic regression, to develop final scores (see Chapter Six for a discussion of logistic regression).

- **Data requirements:** The data source used is medical records, which require data abstraction by trained personnel. A glossary of MedisGroups terms and guidelines for chart abstraction are available.

The MedisGroups scoring system is based on risk factors called "key clinical findings" (KCFs). KCFs indicate abnormalities using physical examination, laboratory, radiological, pathological, and diagnostic test findings. Some key clinical findings are

- Low white blood cell count;

- Low sodium;

- Malignant tumor;

- Pulmonary embolism;

- Bleeding; and

- Complex fracture.

Originally, there were approximately 550 KCFs but this number has been reduced by more than half. Each KCF is linked to one of three "severity groups" that is associated with the likelihood of organ failure. Group 3 indicates the most serious clinical abnormalities. Nearly one-third of the potential 260 KCFs usually are assigned to severity group 0, which will not contribute to the severity rating. Scoring is based on the number and grouping of KCFs present. Iezzoni and Moskowitz (1988) found that, using a MedisGroups-member hospital's data base of patients age 65 and older, nearly 60 percent of those patients with admission scores of 4 died in-hospital compared to less than 1 percent with admission scores of 0 or 1.

When MedisGroups was first being developed, clinicians were consulted to derive the KCFs and their associated severity group. Since then, there has been a shift away from relying on physicians' judgments about relationships between KCFs and the probability of organ failure or mortality in favor of empirical data about these relationships (Steen et al., 1993). A revised version of MedisGroups explicitly includes age in the model, which was found to be a significant predictor of mortality for many of the 64 conditions examined (Iezzoni et al., 1992). Currently, the updating and revision of MedisGroups focus on assessing which KCFs are most predictive of mortality for certain disease groups, since MedisGroups has been criticized for its generic approach. Specifically, the severity group assignment to a KCF is not determined by disease, disease group, or age group (Steen et al., 1993). Finally, although MedisGroups data reporting has been mandated in hospitals in Pennsylvania, Iowa, and Colorado as previously mentioned, the California Office of Statewide Health Planning and Development decided that MedisGroups and other existing severity-adjustment systems to evaluate quality of care were insufficient and mandated a general approach, which requires development of a new system for each condition under study (Johns, 1992).

Computerized Severity Index

The CSI was developed from the Severity of Illness Index (SOII), a manual system intended to link severity and resource use (Horn, 1981; Horn et al., 1985a, 1985b, Horn et al., 1986). The SOII was a generic system and scoring required a variety of clinical judgments. Therefore, the SOII was revised and became the CSI (Iezzoni and Daley, 1992). The key components of the CSI include

- **Outcome(s):** The outcome of interest is length of stay. The population included all persons hospitalized, but it is possible to focus on those admitted for a specific condition or procedure.

- **Severity measure:** Severity is defined as the treatment difficulty presented to physicians, but length of stay is used as a proxy. In other words, clinical factors associated with longer lengths of stay are assigned higher severity levels. For a specific condition, similar risk factors (e.g., hemoglobin and hematocrit) are grouped into larger categories such as hematology.

- **Diagnosis specific:** There are more than 820 disease groups, which are defined by ICD-9-CM codes.

- **Scoring system:** Scores range from a low of 1 (normal to mild) to a high of 4 (life-threatening). Clinical judgment is necessary to complete scoring. Software is available that prompts the user to respond to a series of questions about clinical variables. Hard-copy forms are available for use that can then be entered into a computer at a later time.

- **Data requirements:** The data source used is the medical record, which requires data abstraction. Again, clinicians or trained data abstractors are needed. The CSI depends on ICD-9-CM codes and therefore knowledge of this classification system is necessary.

The CSI has been designed to allow for severity adjustment of health outcomes as a screen for quality of care but also as a system to risk-adjust predictions of resource use. The ability of the CSI to meet these two goals is still in question. A few studies have demonstrated the ability of the CSI to predict resource use, but a study of the CSI that involved using the system to assess hospital care showed that differences might arise because of the way quality problems are defined as well as the condition under study (Iezzoni et al., 1992).

Table 9.6 summarizes the key components of each hospital-based severity-adjustment system.

The major differences between the original MedisGroups system and CSI are the outcome of interest and whether the system is disease-specific or generic. Unfortunately, both systems are subjective and expensive, because they rely on medical record abstraction. Specifically, MedisGroups focuses on in-hospital mortality, which is heavily influenced by discharge policies and it has been recommended that it be replaced by 30-day postadmission mortality (Jencks, Williams, and Kay, 1988). Similarly, the ability to use length of stay as a proxy for treatment difficulty or as a health outcome is still in question. Iezzoni (1989) suggests that once potential severity-adjustment systems have been identified, it may be necessary to apply each system to a sample of medical cases to enable a complete understanding of each approach and its ability to discriminate between groups likely to have good or bad outcomes. Hadorn et al. (1993) developed a set of criteria that vendors of severity-adjustment systems should meet to allow consumers to evaluate them intelligently. Previous criticism of MedisGroups led to the introduction of a revised version that not only is empirically based (i.e., clinical judgments about the relationship between a clinical indicator and in-hospital mortality are no longer needed) but also disease-specific (Steen et al., 1993). Both of these changes are improvements, according

Table 9.6

Comparison of Two Hospital-Based Severity-Adjustment Systems

System Name	MedisGroups	CSI
Outcomes	In-hospital mortality	Length of stay
Patient population	All hospitalized patients	All hospitalized patients
Definition of severity	Risk of imminent organ failure	Treatment difficulty presented to physicians
Disease specific/ generic	Generic	Disease specific
Scoring system	Overall severity is based on a 0 to 4 score on admission and a morbidity score at mid-stay review; clinical judgment is used to assign scores, but a revised version is available based on empirical modeling	Overall severity is scored from 1 to 4; clinical judgment is used to assign scores
Data requirements	Medical chart abstraction; guidelines and a glossary are available	Medical chart abstraction; software and hard copy forms are available

to the criteria of Hadorn and colleagues (1993). These changes highlight the importance of identifying system updates, because many revisions are substantial. The ability of either system to address quality concerns is still being studied. Therefore, anyone seriously considering either of these systems will need to specifically evaluate each one in relation to the specific study question using the criteria of Iezzoni (1989) and Hadorn et al. (1993). This last task is likely to require the input of experts in the field.

Managed Health Care Association Outcomes Management System Project

The Johns Hopkins University asthma severity system is being developed as part of the Managed Health Care Association Outcomes Management System Project (Steinwachs et al., 1995). The purpose of this project is to learn about variations in asthma care, to evaluate the effect of these differences on patients' lives, and to use this knowledge to improve the quality of asthma care. The patient survey includes items for health status and quality of life, number and frequency of symptoms, asthma treatments, and satisfaction with care. Severity was classified based on the symptom that a patient experienced with the greatest frequency. The key components of this system include:

- **Outcome(s):** The outcomes of interest are health status, patient knowledge, and patient satisfaction with care. The system was tested on adult patients with a diagnosis of asthma.

- **Severity measure:** Asthma severity is defined using an international classification scheme. Classifications are based on the greatest frequency reported for any one of the following: chest tightness, wheezing, shortness of breath, occurrence of nocturnal symptoms, and persistence or chronicity of symptoms between asthma attacks.

- **Diagnosis specific:** The survey items used to determine disease severity are specific to asthma, but generic measures are used to assess health status.

- **Scoring system:** Disease severity is rated by both physicians and patients, using ratings of mild, moderate, and severe.

- **Data requirements:** Surveys of patients and physicians (relatively brief) are necessary to gather the required information.

An initial baseline survey of 6,612 adult patients with asthma receiving care in one of 16 managed care organizations found that 13 percent of patients had mild asthma, 45 percent moderate, and 42 percent severe according to the described classification scheme. Physician reports classified few patients as severe compared to classification based on patient reports, but both were strongly associated with health status measures, such as use of inhaled corticosteroids or canceling usual activities.

Type II Diabetes Patient Outcomes Research Team Project

The severity-adjustment system developed by Greenfield et al. (1995) as part of the Type II Diabetes Patient Outcomes Research Team (PORT) project is designed to provide adjustment for ambulatory conditions when functional status is the main outcome of interest. This system is based largely on patient-reported symptoms and responses, which were collected as part of the Type II Diabetes PORT project. The key components of this system include:

- **Outcome(s):** Physical functioning, role functioning, mental health status, disability days within the past six months, physician visits within the past six months, and hospitalizations within the past six months. The system was tested on adult patients with Type II diabetes.

- **Severity measure:** Severity is defined by the total disease burden as evaluated using 15 *body-system-disease measures* including hypertension, lower gastrointestinal disease, and chronic obstructive pulmonary disease. Within each body-system-disease measure are several risk factors that are classified according to whether the factor is part of a diagnosis (e.g., emphysema or asthma), manifestation (e.g., pneumonia or flu with coughing) or symptom (e.g., sputum production or shortness of breath). Conditions related to diabetes are incorporated into the relevant body-system-disease measure (e.g., nephropathy would be categorized under the body-system-disease measure *renal disease*).

- **Generic:** This measure is generic in the sense that it attempts to classify patients according to their total disease burden, which is the aggregate of all conditions or problems each weighted by their severity, but the system has thus far been tested only on patients included in the Type II Diabetes PORT project.

- **Scoring system:** An overall numerical measure of severity (ranges from –22 to 77) is generated but the score can be grouped into descriptive categories that include least, minimal, moderate, and severe. This global measure is constructed by weighting each of 15 conditions. Weights were derived by clinicians according to the expected effect of each disease group on functional status and disability and were tested empirically using regression techniques (see Chapter Six for a discussion of regression analysis).

- **Data requirements:** Administration of a questionnaire that includes items about functional status, symptoms, utilization of services, and other health and health-care-related services is necessary.

Table 9.7 provides a brief comparison of the two ambulatory systems described.

These two systems are significantly different from one another and the asthma severity system is unlikely to be applicable to other conditions without extensive revision, although the framework of the study might be useful to those interested in the quality of ambulatory care and patient satisfaction. The generic severity-adjustment system developed by Greenfield et al. (1995) is more broadly defined, but again, it has not been tested on a random sample of all ambulatory patients, so its generalizability to conditions other than Type II diabetes is still in question. As previously mentioned, application of severity-adjustment techniques to ambulatory conditions is relatively new. A specific

Table 9.7

Comparison of Two Ambulatory-Based Severity-Adjustment Systems

System Name	Managed Health Care Association Outcomes Management System Project	Type II Diabetes PORT Project
Outcomes	Health status, patient knowledge, and patient satisfaction with care	Current physical functioning, role functioning, mental health status; disability days, doctor visits, and hospitalizations in the last six months
Patient population	Adult patients with asthma; patients from 16 managed care organizations were sampled	Patients receiving ambulatory care for diabetes
Definition of severity	Severity classification based on the single asthma symptom that a patient experiences with the greatest frequency	Severity is based on a weighted average of 15 conditions that attempts to describe the total disease burden
Disease specific/ generic	Disease specific	Generic, although the system was developed as part of the Type II Diabetes PORT project and therefore may best be suited to Type II diabetics or other patients with chronic disease
Scoring system	Asthma severity is rated by both physicians and patients, using ratings of mild, moderate, and severe	Severity is derived using clinical judgment and computer modeling; the resulting global score ranges from –22 to 77 and can be grouped into four descriptive categories (least, minimal, moderate, severe)
Data requirements	Administration of surveys to patients and physicians (relatively brief) with subsequent data entry and analysis	Administration of detailed patient surveys with subsequent data entry and analysis

system suitable for the study question of interest may not be available, but prior work can provide insight into how a new system might be developed and what problems to expect.

Severity adjustment of health outcomes is necessary so that valid comparisons can be made, and possibly more important, so that financially costly decisions are avoided. When approaching any study involving health outcomes, you must define the study question as completely as possible and then assess whether severity adjustment is necessary. If severity adjustment is required, you will have to assess the risk factors and data sources needed as well as any potentially applicable existing severity-adjustment systems.

Finally, as this entire chapter demonstrates, a large amount of research is being conducted to improve current severity- and risk-adjustment methods. Anyone who is planning to use one or both techniques is strongly encouraged to seek the advice of experts in the field.

Aday, L. A., *Designing and Conducting Health Surveys: A Comprehensive Guide*, San Francisco, CA: Jossey-Bass Inc., 1989.

Aday, Lu Ann, Charles E. Begley, David R. Lairson, and Carl H. Slater, *Evaluating the Medical Care System: Effectiveness, Efficiency, Equity*, Ann Arbor, MI: Health Administration Press, 1993.

Advisory Committee on Immunization Practices (ACIP), "Update: Pneumococcal Polysaccharide Vaccine Usage—United States," *MMWR*, 33(20):273–281, 1984.

Aldrich, J. H., and F. D. Nelson, *Linear Probability, Logit, and Probit Models*, Beverly Hills, CA: Sage Publications, 1984.

American College of Obstetricians and Gynecologists (ACOG), Task Force on Quality Assurance, *Quality Assurance in Obstetrics and Gynecology*, Washington, DC, 1989.

American College of Obstetricians and Gynecologists, *Quality Assessment and Improvement in Obstetrics and Gynecology*, Washington, DC, 1994.

Andersen, R. M., A. L. Giachello, and L. A. Aday, "Access of Hispanics to Health Care and Cuts in Services: A State-of-the-Art Overview," *Public Health Reports*, 10(3):101(3):238–252, 1986.

Anderson, G. M., R. Brook, and A. Williams, "A Comparison of Cost-Sharing Versus Free Care in Children: Effects on the Demand for Office-Based Medical Care," *Med Care*, 29(9):890–898, 1991.

Anderson, L. M., and D. S. May, "Has the Use of Cervical, Breast, and Colorectal Cancer Screening Increased in the United States?" *American Journal of Public Health*, 85(6):840–842, June 1995.

Arden, N. H., et al., "Prevention and Control of Influenza: Part 1, Vaccines—Recommendations of the Advisory Committee on Immunization Practices (ACIP)," *MMWR*, 42 (RR-6):1–14, 1993.

Ash, A., F. Porell, L. Gruenberg, et al., "Adjusting Medicare Capitation Payments Using Prior Hospitalization," *Health Care Financing Review*, 10(4):17–29, 1989.

Ayanian, J. Z., and A. M. Epstein, "Differences in the Use of Procedures Between Women and Men Hospitalized for Coronary Heart Disease," *New Engl J Med*, 325(4):221–225, 1991.

Babbie, E., *Survey Research Methods*, Belmont, CA: Wadsworth Publishing Company, Inc., 1973.

Babbie, E., *The Practice of Social Research* (3rd ed.), Belmont, CA: Wadsworth Publishing Company, Inc., 1983.

Bailar, J. C., and F. Mosteller, *Medical Uses of Statistics* (2nd ed.), Boston: New England Journal of Medicine Books, 1992.

Bailey, K. D., *Methods of Social Research* (3rd ed.), New York: The Free Press, 1987.

Baker, D. W., C. D. Stevens, and R. H. Brook, "Regular Source of Ambulatory Care and Medical Care Utilization by Patients Presenting to a Public Hospital Emergency Department," *JAMA*, 271(24):1909–1912, 1994.

Ballard, D. J., J. A. Etchason, L. H. Hilborne, et al., *Abdominal Aortic Aneurysm Surgery: A Literature Review and Ratings of Appropriateness and Necessity*, Santa Monica, CA: RAND, JRA-04, 1992.

Barnett, H. J., "Progress in Stroke Prevention: An Overview," *Health Reports*, 6(1):132–138, 1994.

Bates, A. S., J. F. Fitzgerald, R. S. Dittus, and F. D. Wolinsky, "Risk Factors for Underimmunization in Poor Urban Infants," *JAMA*, 272(14):1105–1110, 1994.

Behn, R. D., and J. W. Vaupel, *Quick Analysis for Busy Decision Makers*, New York: Basic Books, 1982.

Bell, R. M., J. Keesey, and T. Richards, "The Urge to Merge: Linking Vital Statistics Records and Medicaid Claims," *Med Care*, 32(10):1004–1018, 1994.

Berk, M. L., and A. C. Monheit, "Data Watch: The Concentration of Health Expenditures: An Update," *Health Affairs*, 145–149, 1992.

Bernstein, S. J., E. A. McGlynn, A. L. Siu, et al., "The Appropriateness of Hysterectomy: A Comparison of Care in Seven Health Plans," *JAMA*, 269:2398–2402, 1993.

Berwick, D. M., and D. L. Wald, "Hospital Leaders' Opinions of the HCFA Mortality Data," *JAMA*, 263:247–249, 1990.

Bigos, S., O. Bowyer, G. Braen, et al., *Acute Low Back Problems in Adults. Clinical Practice Guideline No. 14*, AHCPR Publ. No. 95-0642, Rockville, MD: Agency for Health Care Policy and Research, Public Health Service, U.S. Department of Health and Human Services, December 1994.

Billi, J. E., C. G. Wise, S. I. Sher, et al., "Selection in a Preferred Provider Organization Enrollment," *Health Services Research*, 28(5):563–575, 1993.

Blankenhorn, D. H., et al., "Beneficial Effects of Combined Colestipol-Niacin Therapy on Coronary Atherosclerosis and Coronary Venous Bypass Grafts," *JAMA*, 257:3233–3240, 1987.

Blumberg, M. S., "Risk Adjusting Health Care Outcomes: A Methodologic Review," *Medical Care Review*, 43(2):351–393, Fall 1986.

Blumberg, M. S., "Biased Estimates of Expected Acute Myocardial Infarction Mortality Using MedisGroups Admission Severity Groups," *JAMA*, 265(22):2965–2970, 1991.

Bowen, B., and E. Slavin, "Adjusting Contributions to Address Selection Bias: Three Models for Employers," *Advances in Economics and Health Services Research*, 12:77–96, 1991.

Browner, W. S., "Preventable Complications of Diabetes Mellitus," *Western J Med*, 145:701–703, 1986.

Brunette, M. G., L. Lands, and L. P. Thibodeau, "Childhood Asthma: Prevention of Attacks with Short-Term Corticosteroid Treatment of Upper Respiratory Tract Infection," *Pediatrics*, 81:624–629, 1988.

Buchmueller, T. C., and P. J. Feldstein, "The Effect of Price on Switching Among Health Plans," unpublished paper, June 1995.

Bureau of the Census, *Statistical Abstract of the United States, 1994*, Washington, DC: U.S. Department of Commerce, September 1994.

Campbell, S., and J. Stanley, *Experimental and Quasi-experimental Design for Research*, Chicago, IL: Rand McNally, 1963.

Carlisle D. M., R. Burciaga Valdez, M. F. Shapiro, and R. H. Brook, "Geographic Variation in Rates of Selected Surgical Procedures Within Los Angeles County," *Health Services Research*, 30:27–42, 1995.

Carlisle, D. M., B. D. Leake, and M. F. Shapiro, "Racial and Ethnic Disparities in the Use of Cardiovascular Procedures: Associations with Type of Health Insurance," *American Journal of Public Health*, 82(2):263–267, February 1997.

Carter, G. M., J. P. Newhouse, and D. A. Relles, "How Much Change in the Case Mix Index Is DRG Creep?" *Journal of Health Economics*, 9(4):411–428, 1990.

Centers for Disease Control and Prevention (CDC), "Vaccination Coverage of 2-year Old Children—United States, 1991–1992," *MMWR*, 42:985–988, 1994a.

Centers for Disease Control and Prevention, *Vital and Health Statistics, National Hospital Discharge Survey: Annual Summary, 1992*, Series 13: Data from the National Health Survey, No. 119, DHHS Pub. No. (PHS) 94-1779, Hyattsville, MD: U.S. Department of Health and Human Services, October 1994b.

Centers for Disease Control and Prevention, "Rates of Cesarean Delivery—United States, 1993," *MMWR*, 44(15):303–308, 1995.

Centers for Disease Control and Prevention, "Mortality Patterns—Preliminary Data, 1996," *MMWR*, 46(40):941–944, October 1997a.

Centers for Disease Control and Prevention, "Pneumococcal and Influenza Vaccination Levels Among Adults Aged $\geq$ 65 Years—United States, 1995," *JAMA*, 278(16):1306–1307, 1997b.

Centers for Disease Control and Prevention/National Center for Health Statistics, *1989 Summary: National Hospital Discharge Survey, Advance Data*, No. 199, April 4, 1991.

Centers for Disease Control and Prevention/National Center for Health Statistics, "Current Estimates from the National Health Interview Survey, 1992," *Vital and Health Statistics*, Series 10, No. 189, January 1994a.

Centers for Disease Control and Prevention/National Center for Health Statistics, *National Hospital Ambulatory Medical Care Survey: 1992 Outpatient Department Summary, Advance Data*, No. 248, March 9, 1994b.

Centers for Disease Control and Prevention/National Center for Health Statistics, *Vital and Health Statistics*, Series 10, No. 193, December 1995.

Centers for Disease Control and Prevention/National Center for Health Statistics, *Vital and Health Statistics*, Series 10, No. 194, January 1997a.

Centers for Disease Control and Prevention/National Center for Health Statistics, *Advance Data*, No. 284, May 7, 1997b.

Centers for Disease Control and Prevention/National Center for Health Statistics, *Advance Data*, No. 291, September 1997c.

Centers for Disease Control and Prevention/National Center for Health Statistics website, *Detail Files (1989–95)*, http://www.cdc.gov/nchswww/products/catalogs/subject/natality/natality.htm#1995, 1998.

Chatfield, C., *The Analysis of Time Series: An Introduction* (4th ed.), London: Chapman and Hall, 1989.

Chatfield, C., and A. J. Collins, *Introduction to Multivariate Analysis*, London: Chapman and Hall, 1980.

Chyba, M. M., and L. R. Washington, *Questionnaires from the National Health Interview Survey, 1985–89*, Centers for Disease Control and Prevention/ National Center for Health Statistics, *Vital and Health Statistics*, 1(31), 1993.

Cochran, W. G., *Sampling Techniques* (3rd ed.), New York: John Wiley & Sons, 1977.

Collins, J. G., *Prevalence of Selected Chronic Conditions: United States, 1979–81*, *Vital and Health Statistics*, 10(155), DHHS Publ. No. (PHS)86-1583, July 1986.

Collins, J. G., *Prevalence of Selected Chronic Conditions: United States, 1986–88*, *Vital and Health Statistics*, 10(182), DHHS Publ. No. (PHS)93-1510, February 1993.

Cook, T., and S. Campbell, *Quasi-experimentation*, Chicago, IL: Rand McNally, 1979.

Cornelius, E., J. Feldman, J. A. Marsteller, and K. Liu, "Creating a MEDPAR Analog to the RUG-III Classification System," *Health Care Financing Review*, 16(2):101–126, 1994.

Daley, J., "Criteria by Which to Evaluate Risk-Adjusted Outcomes Programs in Cardiac Surgery," *Annals of Thoracic Surgery*, 58:1827–1835, 1994.

Davidson, B. N., S. Sofaer, and P. Gertler, "Consumer Information and Biased Selection in the Demand for Coverage Supplementing Medicare," *Soc Sci Med*, 34(9):1023–1034, 1992.

Davies, A. R., and J. E. Ware, Jr., *GHAA's Consumer Satisfaction Survey and User's Manual* (2nd ed.), Washington, DC: The Group Health Association of America, 1991.

Davis, K., and D. Rowland, "Uninsured and Underserved: Inequities in Health Care in the United States," *Milbank Memorial Fund Quarterly*, 61(2):149–176, 1983.

Dawber, T. R., *The Framingham Study: The Epidemiology of Atherosclerotic Disease*, Cambridge, MA: Harvard University Press, 1980.

DCCT Research Group, "The Effect of Intensive Treatment of Diabetes on the Development and Progression of Long-Term Complications in Insulin-Dependent Diabetes Mellitus," *New Engl J Med*, 329(14):977–986, 1993.

DeFriese, G. H., A. T. Evans, T. C. Ricketts, and E. P. Cromartie, *North Carolina Medical Society Practice Variation Study of Hysterectomy*, Chapel Hill, NC: University of North Carolina, 1989.

Depression Guideline Panel, *Depression in Primary Care: Volume 1, Detection and Diagnosis. Clinical Practice Guideline, No. 5,* AHCPR Publ. No. 93-0550, Rockville, MD: Agency for Health Care Policy and Research, Public Health Service, U.S. Department of Health and Human Services, April 1993a.

Depression Guideline Panel, *Depression in Primary Care: Volume 2, Treatment of Major Depression. Clinical Practice Guideline, No. 5,* AHCPR Publ. No. 93-0551, Rockville, MD: Agency for Health Care Policy and Research, Public Health Service, U.S. Department of Health and Human Services, April 1993b.

Diehr, P., C. W. Madden, A. Cheadle, et al., "Estimating County Percentages of People without Health Insurance," *Inquiry,* 28:413–419, 1991.

Diehr, P., C. W. Madden, D. P. Martin, et al., "Who Enrolled in a State Program for the Uninsured: Was There Adverse Selection?" *Med Care,* 31(12):1093–1105, 1993.

Dillman, D. A., *Mail and Telephone Surveys: The Total Design Method,* New York: John Wiley & Sons, 1978.

Dobson, A. J., *An Introduction to Generalized Linear Models,* London: Chapman and Hall, 1990.

Donaldson, M. S., and K. N. Lohr (eds.), *Health Data in the Information Age,* Washington, DC: National Academy Press, 1994.

Doyle, J. C., "Unnecessary Hysterectomies: Study of 6248 Operations in Thirty-Five Hospitals during 1948," *JAMA,* 151:360–365, 1953.

Draper, N., and H. Smith, *Applied Regression Analysis* (2nd ed.), New York: John Wiley & Sons, 1981.

Dubois, R. W., R. H. Brook, and W. H. Rogers, "Adjusted Hospital Death Rates: A Potential Screen for Quality of Medical Care," *AJPH,* 77:1162–1166, 1987.

Dyck, F. J., F. A. Murphy, and J. K. Murphy, "Effect of Surveillance on the Number of Hysterectomies in the Province of Saskatchewan," *New Engl J Med,* 296:1326–1328, 1977.

Early Treatment Diabetic Retinopathy Study Research Group, "Photocoagulation for Diabetic Macular Edema: Early Treatment Diabetic Retinopathy Study Report No. 1," *Arch Ophthalmol,* 103:1796–1806, 1985.

Edwards, N., D. Honeman, D. Burley, and M. Navarro, "Refinement of the Medicare Diagnosis-Related Groups to Incorporate a Measure of Severity," *Health Care Financing Review,* 16(2):45–64, 1994.

Ellis, R. P., and T. G. McGuire, "Supply-Side and Demand-Side Cost Sharing in Health Care," *Journal of Economic Perspectives,* 7(4):135–151, 1993.

Farley, D. O., J. D. Kallich, G. M. Carter, et al., *Designing a Capitation Payment Plan for Medicare End Stage Renal Disease Services*, Santa Monica, CA: RAND, MR-391-HCFA, 1994.

Feigl, P., G. Glaefke, L. Ford, et al., "Studying Patterns of Cancer Care: How Useful Is the Medical Record?" *American Journal of Public Health*, 78(5):526–533, 1988.

Finkler, M. D., and D. D. Wirtschaftler, "Cost-Effectiveness and Obstetric Services," *Med Care*, 29:951–963, 1991.

Flamm, B. L., O. W. Lim, C. Jones, et al., "Vaginal Birth After Cesarean Section: Results of a Multicenter Study," *Am J Obstet Gynecol*, 158:1079–1084, 1988.

Fleiss, J. L., *Statistical Methods for Rates and Proportions*, New York: John Wiley & Sons, 1981.

Freedman, D., R. Pisani, R. Purves, and A. Adhikari, *Statistics* (2nd ed.), New York: W. W. Norton & Company, 1991.

Freeman, H. E., R. J. Blendon, L. H. Aiken, et al., "Americans Report on Their Access to Health Care," *Health Affairs*, 6–18, Spring 1987.

Friday, G. A., and P. Fireman, "Morbidity and Mortality of Asthma," *Pediatric Clinics of North America*, 35:1149–1163, 1988.

Friedman, G. D., and J. V. Selby, "Colorectal Cancer: Have We Identified an Effective Screening Strategy?" *J Gen Intern Med*, 5(Suppl):523–527, 1990.

Graves, E. J., *Detailed Diagnoses and Procedures, National Hospital Discharge Survey: United States, 1990, Vital and Health Statistics*, 113(13):118, 1991.

Greenfield, A., L. Sullivan, K. A. Dukes, et al., "Development and Testing of a New Measure of Case Mix for Use in Office Practice," *Med Care*, 33(4):AS47–AS55, 1995.

Greenfield, S., D. M. Blanco, R. M. Elashoff, et al., "Patterns of Care Related to Age of Breast Cancer Patients," *JAMA*, 257:2766–2770, 1987.

Greenfield, S., H. U. Aronow, R. M. Elashoff, and D. Watanabe, "Flaws in Mortality Data: The Hazards of Ignoring Comorbid Disease," *JAMA*, 260(15):2253–2255, 1988.

Greenfield, S., G. Apolone, B. J. McNeil, and P. D. Cleary, "The Importance of Co-Existent Disease in the Occurrence of Postoperative Complications and One-Year Recovery in Patients Undergoing Total Hip Replacement: Comorbidity and Outcomes after Hip Replacement," *Med Care*, 31(2):141–154, 1993.

Gross, P. A., et al., "Association of Influenza Immunization with Reduction in Mortality in an Elderly Population: A Prospective Study," *Arch Intern Med*, 148:562–565, 1988.

Groves, R. M., and R. L. Kahn, *Surveys by Telephone: A National Comparison with Personal Interviews*, New York: Academic Press, Inc., 1979.

Haas, J. S., I. S. Udvarhelyi, C. N. Morris, and A. M. Epstein, "The Effect of Providing Health Coverage to Poor Uninsured Pregnant Women in Massachusetts," *JAMA*, 269:87–91, 1993.

Hadorn, D. C., E. B. Keeler, W. H. Rogers, and R. H. Brook, *Assessing the Performance of Mortality Prediction*, Santa Monica, CA: RAND, MR-181-HCFA, 1993.

Hannan, E. L., H. Kilburn, H. Bernard, et al., "Coronary Artery Bypass Surgery: The Relationship Between Inhospital Mortality and Surgical Volume After Controlling for Clinical Risk Factors," *Med Care*, 29(11):1094–1107, 1991.

Hannan E. L., D. T. Arani, L. W. Johnson, et al, "Percutaneous Transluminal Coronary Angioplasty in New York State," *JAMA*, 268(21):3092–3097, 1992a.

Hannan, E. L., H. Kilburn, Jr., J. F. O'Donnell, et al., "Adult Open Heart Surgery in New York State," *JAMA*, 264:2768–2774, 1990.

Hannan, E. L., H. Kilburn, Jr., M. L. Lindsey, and R. Lewis, "Clinical Versus Administrative Data Bases for CABG Surgery: Does It Matter?" *Med Care*, 30(10):892–907, 1992b.

Hannan, E. L., H. Kilburn, M. Racz, et al., "Improving the Outcomes of Coronary Artery Bypass Surgery in New York State," *JAMA*, 271(10):761–766, 1994.

Hays, R. D., C. D. Sherbourne, and R. M. Mazel, RAND 36-Item Health Survey 1.0, Santa Monica, DA: RAND RP-247, 1993 (also available online: www.sf-36.com/).

Haynes, R. B., D. W. Taylor, D. L. Sackett, et al., "Prevention of Functional Impairment by Endarterectomy for Symptomatic High-Grade Carotid Stenosis, North American Symptomatic Carotid Endarterectomy Trial Collaborators," *JAMA*, 271(16):1256–1259, 1994.

Hays, R. D., K. B. Wells, C. D. Sherbourne, et al., "Functioning and Well-Being Outcomes of Patients with Depression Compared with Chronic General Medical Illnesses," *Arch Gen Psych*, 52:11–19, 1995.

Herbert, P. R., et al., "The Community-Based Randomized Trials of Pharmacologic Treatment for Mild-to-Moderate Hypertension," *Am J Epidemiology*, 127:581–590, 1988.

Higgins, T. L., F. G. Estafanous, F. D. Loop, et al., "Stratification of Morbidity and Mortality Outcome by Preoperative Risk Factors in Coronary Artery Bypass Patients: A Clinical Severity Score," *JAMA*, 267(17):2344–2348, 1992.

Hilborne, L. H., L. L. Leape, S. J. Bernstein, et al., "The Appropriateness of Use of Percutaneous Transluminal Coronary Angioplasty in New York State," *JAMA*, 269(6):761–765, 1993.

Hill, J. W., and R. S. Brown, *Biased Selection in the TEFRA HMO/CMP Program*, Princeton, NJ: Mathematica Policy Research, MPR-7786-503, 1990.

Hobson, R. W., II, D. G. Weiss, W. S. Fields, et al., "Efficacy of Carotid Endarterectomy for Asymptomatic Carotid Stenosis. The Veterans Affairs Cooperative Study Group," *New Engl J Med*, 328(4):221–227, 1993.

Horn, S. D., "Validity, Reliability and Implications of an Index of Inpatient Severity of Illness," *Med Care*, 19:354–362, 1981.

Horn, S. D., P. D. Sharkey, A. F. Chambers, and R. A. Horn, "Severity of Illness Within DRGs: Impact on Prospective Payment," *Am J Public Health*, 75:1195–1199, 1985a.

Horn, S. D., G. Bulkley, P. D. Sharkey, et al., "Interhospital Differences in Severity of Illness: Problems for Prospective Payment Based on Diagnosis-Related Groups (DRGs)," *N Engl J Med*, 313:20–24, 1985b.

Horn, S. D., R. A. Horn, P. D. Sharkey, and A. F. Chambers, "Severity of Illness Within DRGs: Homogeneity Study," *Med Care*, 24:225–235, 1986.

Hosmer, D. W., and S. Lemeshow, *Applied Logistic Regression*, New York: John Wiley & Sons, 1989.

Iezzoni, L. I., "Using Severity Information for Quality Assessment: A Review of Three Cases by Five Severity Measures," *Quality Review Bulletin*, 376–382, December 1989.

Iezzoni, L. I., "Risk Adjustment for Medical Effectiveness Research: An Overview of Conceptual and Methodological Considerations," *Journal of Investigative Medicine*, 43(2):136–150, 1992.

Iezzoni, L. I. (ed.), *Risk Adjustment for Measuring Health Care Outcomes* (2nd ed.), Ann Arbor, MI: Health Administration Press, 1997.

Iezzoni, L. I., and M. A. Moskowitz, "A Clinical Assessment of MedisGroups," *JAMA*, 260(21):3159–3163, 1988.

Iezzoni, L. I., and J. Daley, "A Description and Clinical Assessment of the Computerized Severity Index," *Quality Review Bulletin*, 44–52, February 1992.

Iezzoni, L. I., M. Shwartz, M. A. Moskowitz, et al., "Illness Severity and Costs of Admissions at Teaching and Non-Teaching Hospitals," *JAMA*, 264(11):1426–1431, 1990.

Iezzoni, L. I., M. Schwartz, and J. Restuccia, "The Role of Severity Information in Current Health Policy Debates: A Survey of State and Regional Concerns," *Inquiry*, 28:117, 1991.

Iezzoni, L. I., A. S. Ash, G. A. Coffman, and M. A. Moskowitz, "Predicting In-Hospital Mortality: A Comparison of Severity Adjustment Approaches," *Med Care*, 30(4):347–359, 1992.

Iezzoni, L. I., B. A. Hotchkin, A. Ash, et al., "MedisGroups Data Bases: The Impact of Data Collection Guidelines on Predicting In-Hospital Mortality," *Med Care*, 31(3):277–283, 1993.

Iezzoni, L. I., M. Shwartz, A. S. Ash, et al., "Risk Adjustment Methods Can Affect Perceptions of Outcomes," *Risk and Outcomes*, 9(2):43–48, Summer 1994.

Jencks, S. F., D. K. Williams, and T. L. Kay, "Assessing Hospital-Associated Deaths from Discharge Data: The Role of Length of Stay and Comorbidities," *JAMA*, 260(15):2240–2246, 1988.

Jenkins, V. R., "Unnecessary—Elective—Indicated? Audit Criteria of the American College of Obstetricians and Gynecologists to Assess Abdominal Hysterectomy for Uterine Leiomyoma," *Qual Rev Bull*, 3:7–12,21, 1977.

Johns, L., "Measuring Quality in California," *Health Affairs*, 11(1):266–270, Spring 1992.

Johnson, R. A., and D. W. Wichern, *Applied Multivariate Statistical Analysis*, Englewood Cliffs: Prentice Hall, 1988.

Kahn, K. L., W. H. Rogers, L. V. Rubenstein, et al., "Measuring Quality of Care with Explicit Process Criteria Before and After Implementation of the DRG-Based Prospective Payment System," *JAMA*, 264(15):1969–1973, 1990.

Kahn, K. L., D. Draper, E. B. Keeler, et al., *The Effects of the DRG-Based Prospective Payment System on Quality of Care for Hospitalized Medicare Patients*, Santa Monica: CA, RAND, R-3931-HCFA, 1992.

Keeler, E. B., "What Proportion of Hospital Cost Differences Is Justifiable?" *Journal of Health Economics*, 9:359–364, 1990.

Keeler, E. B., *Causes and Effects of Expensive Hospitalizations*, Santa Monica, CA: RAND, N-3205-HCFA, 1991.

Keeler, E. B., et al., "Changes in Sickness at Admission Following the Introduction of the Prospective Payment System," in *A Summary of the Effects of DRG-*

Based Prospective Payment System on Quality of Care for Hospitalized Medicare Patients, Santa Monica, CA: RAND, N-3132-HCFA, October 1990.

Kelsey, J. L., and S. Hoffman, "Risk Factors for Hip Fracture," *N Engl J Med*, 316:404–406, 1987.

Kish, L., *Statistical Design for Research*, New York: John Wiley & Sons, 1987.

Kish, L., *Survey Sampling*, New York: John Wiley & Sons, 1965.

Kleinman, L. C., et al. "The Medical Appropriateness of Tympanostomy Tubes Proposed for Children Younger Than 16 Years in the United States," *JAMA*, 271(16):1250–1265, 1994.

Konstam, M., K. Dracup, D. Baker, et al., *Heart Failure: Evaluation and Care of Patients with Left-Ventricular Systolic Dysfunction. Clinical Practice Guideline No. 11*, AHCPR Publ. No. 94-0612, Rockville, MD: Agency for Health Care Policy and Research, Public Health Service, U.S. Department of Health and Human Services, June 1994.

Kottke, T. E., et al., "Attributes of Successful Smoking Cessation Interventions in Medical Practice: A Meta-Analysis of 39 Controlled Trials," *JAMA*, 259:2883–2889, 1988.

Koutsoyiannis, A., *Theory of Econometrics: An Introductory Exposition of Econometric Methods* (2nd ed.), London: The MacMillan Press Ltd., 1985.

Kronick R., Z. Zhou, and T. Dreyfus, "Making Risk Adjustment Work for Everyone," *Inquiry*, 32:41–55, Spring 1995.

Krumholtz, H. M., et al., "Lack of Association Between Cholesterol and Coronary Heart Disease Mortality and Morbidity and All-Cause Mortality in Persons Older Than 70 years," *JAMA*, 272(12):1335–1340, 1994.

Leape, L. L., L. H. Hilborne, R. E. Park, et al., "The Appropriateness of Use of Coronary Artery Bypass Graft Surgery in New York State," *JAMA*, 269(6):753–760, 1993.

Lee, P. P., C. J. Kamberg, L. H. Hilborne, et al., *Cataract Surgery: A Literature Review and Ratings of Appropriateness and Cruciality*, Santa Monica, CA: RAND, JRA-06, 1993.

Levy, P. S., and S. Lemeshow, *Sampling of Populations: Methods and Applications*, New York: John Wiley & Sons, 1991.

Lilford, R. J., H. A. Van Coeverden De Groot, P. H. Moore, and P. Bingham, "The Relative Risk of Cesarean Section and Vaginal Delivery: A Detailed Analysis to Exclude the Effects of Medical Disorders and Other Acute Pre-existing Physiological Disturbances," *Br J Obstet Gynaecol*, 97:883–892, 1990.

Little, R.J.A., and D. B. Rubin, *Statistical Analysis with Missing Data*, New York: John Wiley & Sons, 1987.

Lohr, Kathleen N. (ed.), *Medicare: A Strategy for Quality Assurance*, Washington, DC: National Academy Press, 1990.

Luft, H. S., and E. Morrison, "Alternate Delivery Systems," in E. Ginzberg (ed.), *Health Services Research: Key to Health Policy*, Cambridge, MA: Harvard University Press, 1991.

Lui, K. J., et al., "Impact of Influenza Epidemics on Mortality in the United States from October 1972 to May 1985," *American Journal of Public Health*, 77(6):712–716, 1987.

Mansfield, E., *Statistics for Business and Economics: Methods and Applications* (4th ed.), New York: W. W. Norton and Company, 1991.

Marre, M., et al., "Prevention of Diabetic Nephropathy with Enalapril in Iormotensive Diabetics with Macroalbuminuria," *Br Med J*, 297:1092–1095, 1988.

Mausner, J. S., and S. Kramer, *Epidemiology: An Introductory Text*, Philadelphia, PA: W. B. Saunders Company, 1985.

Mazze, R. S., et al., "An Epidemiological Model for Diabetes Mellitus in the United States: Five Major Complications," *Diabetes Res Clin Pract*, 1:185–191, 1985.

McConnell, J. D., M. J. Barry, R. B. Bruskewitz, et al., *Benign Prostatic Hyperplasia: Diagnosis and Treatment. Clinical Practice Guideline, Number 8*, AHCPR Publ. No. 94-0582, Rockville, MD: Agency for Health Care Policy and Research, Public Health Service, U.S. Department of Health and Human Services, February 1994.

McGlynn, E. A., D. Naylor, G. M. Anderson, et al., "Comparison of the Appropriateness of Coronary Angiography and Coronary Artery Bypass Graft Surgery Between Canada and New York State," *JAMA*, 272(12):934–940, 1994.

Michels, K. B., and S. Yusuf, "Does PTCA in Acute Myocardial Infarction Affect Mortality and Reinfarction Rates? A Quantitative Overview (Meta-analysis) of the Randomized Clinical Trials," *Circulation*, 91(2):476–485, 1995.

Miller, J. M., "Maternal and Neonatal Morbidity and Mortality in Cesarean Section," *Obstet Gynecol Clin NA*, 15:629–638, 1988.

Miller, N. F., "Hysterectomy, Therapeutic Necessity or Surgical Racket?" *Am J Obstet Gynecol*, 51:804–810, 1946.

Miller R. G., *Survival Analysis*, New York: John Wiley & Sons, 1981.

Miller, R. H., and H. S. Luft, "Managed Care Plan Performance Since 1980. A Literature Analysis," *JAMA*, 271(19):1512–1519, 1994.

Millman, M. (ed.), *Access to Health Care in America*, Washington, DC: National Academy Press, 1993.

Mitchell, J. B., "Time Trends in Inpatient Physician Spending," *Health Services Research*, 28(5):641–660, 1993.

Moser, C. A., and G. Kalton, *Survey Methods in Social Investigation* (2nd ed.), London: Heinemann Educational, 1971.

Murata, P. J., E. A. McGlynn, A. L. Siu, et al., "Quality Measures for Prenatal Care: A Comparison of Care in Six Health Care Plans," *Arch Fam Med*, 3(1):41–49, 1994.

National Cancer Institute Breast Cancer Screening Consortium, "Screening Mammography: A Missed Clinical Opportunity? Results of the NCI Breast Cancer Screening Consortium and National Health Interview Survey Studies," *JAMA*, 264(1):54–58, 1990.

National Cancer Institute (NCI), *1987 Annual Cancer Statistics Review: Including Cancer Trends: 1950–1985*, Rockville, MD: NIH Publ. 88-2789, Superintendent of Documents, 1988.

National Center for Health Statistics (NCHS), *Prevention Profile, Health, United States 1989*, Hyattsville, MD: Public Health Services, 1990.

National Center for Health Statistics, "Annual Summary of Births, Marriages, Divorces, and Deaths: United States, 1993," *Monthly Vital Statistics Report*, 42(13):1–36, 1994.

National Committee for Quality Assurance (NCQA), *The State of Managed Care Quality*, Washington, DC, October 1, 1997a.

National Committee for Quality Assurance, *A Road Map for Information Systems*, Washington, DC, 1997b.

National Heart, Lung and Blood Institute (NHLBI), "Hypertension Prevalence and the Status of Awareness, Treatment, and Control in the United States: Final Report of the Subcommittee on Definition and Prevalence of the 1984 Joint National Committee," *Hypertension*, 7(3):457–468, 1985.

Neter, J., W. Wasserman, and M. H. Kutner, *Applied Linear Statistical Models: Regression, Analysis of Variance, and Experimental Designs* (3rd ed.), Burr Ridge, IL: Irwin, 1990.

Newhouse, J. P., "Rate Adjusters for Medicare Capitation," *Health Care Financing Review, 1986 Annual Supplement*, HCFA Publication No. 03225, Office of

Research and Demonstrations, Health Care Financing Administration, Washington, DC: U.S. Government Printing Office, December 1986.

Newhouse, J. P., "Economics Analysis: Patients at Risk: Health Reform and Risk Adjustment," *Health Affairs*, 132–146, 1994.

Newhouse, J. P., "Reimbursing Health Plans and Health Providers: Selection vs. Efficiency in Production," unpublished manuscript, 1995.

Newhouse, J. P., and The Insurance Experiment Group, *Free for All? Lessons from the RAND Health Insurance Experiment*, Cambridge, MA: Harvard University Press, 1993.

Newhouse, J. P., et al., "Are Fee-for-Service Costs Increasing Faster Than HMO's Costs?" *Med Care*, 23(8):960–966, 1985.

Newhouse, J. P., W. G. Manning, E. B. Keeler, and E. M. Sloss, "Adjusting Capitation Rates Using Objective Health Measures and Prior Utilization," *Health Care Financing Review*, 10(3), 41–54, Spring 1989.

Newhouse, J. P., W. G. Manning, Jr., E. B. Keeler, and E. M. Sloss, "Risk Adjustment for a Children's Capitation Rate," *Health Care Financing Review*, 15(1):39–54, Fall 1993.

New York State Department of Health, *Coronary Artery Bypass Graft Surgery in New York State*, December 1992.

Oddone, E. Z., P. A. Cowper, J. D. Hamilton, et al., "A Cost-Effectiveness Analysis of Hepatitis B Vaccine in Predialysis Patients," *Health Services Research*, 28(1):97–121, 1993.

Office of Statewide Health Planning and Development, *Report of Results from the OSHPD Reabstracting Project: An Evaluation of the Reliability of Selected Patient Discharge Data, July Through December 1988*, Sacramento, CA: Office of Statewide Health Planning and Development, 1990.

Oldridge, N. B., et al., "Cardiac Rehabilitation after Myocardial Infarction," *JAMA*, 260:945–950, 1988.

Ostrom, C. W., *Time Series Analysis: Regression Techniques*, Beverly Hills, CA: Sage Publications, 1978.

Parcel, G. S., et al., "A Comparison of Absentee Rates of Elementary Schoolchildren with Asthma and Nonasthmatic Schoolmates," *Pediatrics*, 64:878–881, 1979.

Park, R. E., R. H. Brook, J. Kosecoff, et al., "Explaining Variations in Hospital Death Rates: Randomness, Severity of Illness, Quality of Care," *JAMA*, 264(4):484–490, 1990.

Parving, H. H., et al., "Early Aggressive Antihypertensive Treatment Reduces Rate of Decline in Kidney Function in Diabetic Nephropathy," *Lancet*, 1176–1178, May 1983.

Pauly, M. V., *Doctors and Their Workshops*, Chicago: University of Chicago Press, 1980.

Peterson, E. D., L. K. Shaw, E. R. DeLong, D. B. Pryor, R. M. Califf, and D. B. Mark, "Racial Variation in the Use of Coronary Revascularization Procedures: Are the Differences Real? Do They Matter?" *N Engl J Med*, 336(7): 480–486, 1997.

Petitti, D. B., *Methods for Quantitative Synthesis in Medicine*, New York: Oxford University Press, 1994.

Phillips, R. C., and D. J. Lansky, "Outcomes Management in Heart Valve Replacement Surgery: Early Experience," *Journal of Heart Valve Disease*, 1(1):42–50, 1992.

Pindyck, R. S., and D. L. Rubinfeld, *Econometric Models and Economic Forecasts* (3rd ed.), New York: McGraw-Hill, Inc., 1991.

Piper, J. M., W. A. Ray, and M. R. Griffon, "Effects of Medicaid Eligibility Expansion on Prenatal Care and Pregnancy Outcome in Tennessee," *JAMA*, 264:2219–2223, 1990.

The President's Advisory Commission on Consumer Protection and Quality in the Health Care Industry, *Quality First: Better Health Care for All Americans*, final report to the President of the United States, Washington, DC: U.S. Government Printing Office, 1998.

Price, J. R., and J. W. Mays, "Selection and the Competitive Standing of Health Plans in a Multiple-Choice Multiple Insurer Market," in R. M. Scheffler and L. W. Kossiter (eds.), *Advances in Health Economics and Health Services Research*, Volume 6, Greenwich, Connecticut: JAI Press, 1985.

Pryor, D. B., R. M. Califf, F. E. Harrell, Jr., et al., "Clinical Data Bases: Accomplishments and Unrealized Potential," *Med Care*, 23(5):623–647, May 1985.

Riley, G., J. Lubitz, and E. Rabey, "Enrollee Health Status Under Medicare Risk Contracts: An Analysis of Mortality Rates," *Health Services Research*, 26(2):137–163, 1991.

The Robert Wood Johnson Foundation, *Access to Health Care in the United States: Results of a 1986 Survey*, Special Report No. 2, Princeton, NJ, 1987.

Robinson, C. A., W. B. Evans, J. A. Mahanes, and S. J. Sepe, "Progress on the Childhood Immunization Initiative," *Public Health Reports*, 109(5):594–600, 1994.

Robinson, J. C., H. S. Luft, L. B. Gardner, and E. M. Morrison, "A Method for Risk-Adjusting Employer Contributions to Competing Health Insurance Plans," *Inquiry*, 28(2):107–116, 1991.

Romano, P. S., "Can Administrative Data Be Used to Compare the Quality of Health Care," *Medical Care Review*, 50(4):451–477, Winter 1993.

Romm, F. J., and S. M. Putnam, "The Validity of the Medical Record," *Med Care*, 19(3):310–315, 1981.

Roos, L. L., N. P. Roos, and S. M. Shart, "Monitoring Adverse Outcomes of Surgery Using Administrative Data," *Health Care Financing Review* (Annual Suppl.):5–16, 1987.

Roos, N. P., E. Shapiro, and R. Tate, "Does a Small Minority of Elderly Account for a Majority of Health Care Expenditures? A Sixteen-Year Perspective," *The Milbank Quarterly*, 67(3–4):347–369, 1989.

Roos, L. L., N. P. Roos, E. S. Fisher, and T. A. Bubolz, "Strengths and Weaknesses of Health Insurance Data Systems for Assessing Outcomes," in A. C. Gelijns (ed.), *Modern Methods of Clinical Investigation*, Volume 1, Washington, DC: National Academy Press, 1990.

Rossi, P. H., J. D. Wright, and A. B. Anderson (eds.), *Handbook of Survey Research*, San Diego, CA: Academic Press, Inc., 1983.

Russell, L., and C. Manning, "The Effect of Prospective Payment on Medicare Expenditures," *N Eng J Med*, 320:439–444, 1989.

Schappert, S. M., *Office Visits for Otitis Media: US, 1975–90*, Advance Data from *Vital and Health Statistics* (214), U.S. Department of Health and Human Services, 1992.

Selby, J. V., et al., "A Case-Control Study of Screening Sigmoidoscopy and Mortality from Colorectal Cancer," *New Engl J Med*, 326:653–657, 1992.

Siu, A. L., E. A. McGlynn, H. Morgenstern, and R. H. Brook, "A Fair Approach to Comparing Quality of Care," *Health Affairs*, 62–75, Spring 1991.

Siu, A. L., E. A. McGlynn, M. H. Beers, et al., *Choosing Quality-of-Care Measures Based on the Expected Impact of Improved Quality of Care for the Major Causes of Mortality and Morbidity*, Santa Monica, CA: RAND, JR-03, 1992.

Snedecor, G. W., and W. G. Cochran, *Statistical Methods* (7th ed.), Ames: The Iowa State University Press, 1980.

Steen, P. M., A. C. Brewster, R. C. Bradbury, et al., "Predicted Probabilities of Hospital Death as a Measure of Admission Severity of Illness," *Inquiry*, 30:128–141, Summer 1993.

Steinwachs, D. M., A. Wu, E. A. Skinner, and D. Campbell, "Managed Health Care Association Outcomes Management System Project: Asthma Patient Outcomes Study Baseline Survey Summary Report," unpublished manuscript, January 1995.

Stewart, A. L., and J. E. Ware, Jr., *Measuring Functioning and Well-Being: The Medical Outcomes Study Approach*, Durham, NC: Duke University Press, 1992.

Stewart, P. J., C. Dulberg, A. C. Amill, et al., "Diagnosis of Dystocia and Management with Cesarean Section Among Primiparous Women in Ottawa-Carleton," *Can Med Assoc J*, 142(5):459–463, 1990.

Stokey, E., and R. Zeckhauser, *A Primer for Policy Analysis*, New York: W. W. Norton & Company, 1978.

Stool, S. E., A. O. Berg, S. Berman, et al., *Otitis Media with Effusion in Young Children. Clinical Practice Guideline, No. 12*, AHCPR Publ. No. 94-0622, Rockville, MD: Agency for Health Care Policy and Research, Public Health Service, U.S. Department of Health and Human Services, July 1994.

Sudman, S., and N. M. Bradburn, *Asking Questions: A Practical Guide to Questionnaire Design*, San Francisco, CA: Jossey-Bass Inc., 1982.

Swartz, K., "Dynamics of People Without Health Insurance. Don't Let the Numbers Fool You," *JAMA*, 271(1):64–66, 1994.

Swartz, K., "Reducing Risk Selection Requires More Than Risk Adjustments," *Inquiry*, 32(1):6–10, Spring 1995.

Theroux, P., et al., "Aspirin, Heparin, or Both to Treat Acute Unstable Angina," *New Engl J Med*, 319:1105–1111, 1988.

Thomas, C. L., *Taber's Cyclopedic Medical Dictionary*, Edition 15, Philadelphia, PA: F. A. Davis Company, 1981.

Tobacman, J. F., P. P. Lee, B. Zimmerman, H. Kolder, L. Hilborne, and R. H. Brook, "Assessment of the Appropriateness of Cataract Surgery at Ten Academic Medical Centers," *Ophthalmology*, 103:207–215, 1996.

Trevino, F. M., E. Moyer, R. B. Valdez, and C. A. Stromp-Benham, "Health Insurance Coverage and Utilization of Health Services by Mexican Americans, Mainland Puerto Ricans, and Cuban Americans," *JAMA*, 265(2):233–237, 1991.

U.S. Preventive Services Task Force (USPSTF), *Guide to Clinical Preventive Services* (2nd ed.), Baltimore, MD: Williams & Wilkins, 1995.

U. S. Public Health Service, *Healthy People 2000: National Health Promotion and Disease Prevention Objectives,* Department of Health and Human Services, Washington, D.C., 1990.

U.S. Public Health Service, "Childhood Immunizations Gain New Support," *Prevention Report,* Washington, D.C., 1994.

Van de Werf, F., "Thrombolysis for Acute Myocardial Infarction," *Haemostasis,* 24(2):65–68, 1994.

van Vliet, R. C., and W. P. van de Ven, "Towards a Capitation Formula for Competing Health Insurers. An Empirical Analysis," *Soc Sci Med,* 34(9):1035–1048, 1992.

Vistnes, J., *Private Health Insurance Premiums in 1987: Policyholders Under Age 65,* AHCPR Publ. No. 92-0061, National Medical Expenditure Survey Data Summary 5, Rockville, MD: Agency for Health Care Policy and Research, Public Health Service, August 1992.

Wagner, J. L., R. C. Herdman, and S. Wadhwa, "Cost Effectiveness of Colorectal Cancer Screening in the Elderly," *Ann Int Med,* 115(10):807–817, 1991.

Warner, K. E., and B. R. Luce, *Cost-Benefit and Cost-Effectiveness Analysis in Health Care: Principles, Practice, and Potential,* Ann Arbor, MI: Health Administration Press, 1982.

Weiner, J. P., B. H. Starfield, D. M. Steinwachs, and L. M. Mumford, "Development and Application of a Population-Oriented Measure of Ambulatory Care Case-Mix," *Med Care,* 2(5):452–472, 1991.

Weisberg, S., *Applied Linear Regression,* New York: John Wiley & Sons, 1985.

Weisberg, H. F., and B. D. Bowen, *An Introduction to Survey Research and Data Analysis,* San Francisco, CA: W. H. Freeman and Co., 1977.

Welch, H. G., M. E. Miller, and W. P. Welch, "Physician Profiling: An Analysis of Inpatient Practice Patterns in Florida and Oregon," *New Engl J Med,* 330(9):607–612, 1994.

Wennberg, J. E., *A Systematic Study of the Nature, Extent, Causes and Cost Implications of Small Area Variation,* Final Report to the John A. Hartford Foundation, Grant #85163-3H, Hanover, NH: Department of Community and Family Medicine, Dartmouth Medical School, undated.

Wennberg, J. E., N. Roos, L. Sola, et al., "Use of Claims Data Systems to Evaluate Health Care Outcomes: Mortality and Reoperation Following Prostatectomy," *JAMA,* 257(7):933–936, 1987.

Wenneker, M. B., and A. M. Epstein, "Racial Inequalities in the Use of Procedures for Patients with Ischemic Heart Disease in Massachusetts," *JAMA*, 261(2):253–257, 1989.

White House Task Force on Health Risk Pooling, *Health Risk Pooling for Small-Group Health Insurance*, Washington, DC: GPO, 1993.

Wickizer, T., "The Effect of Utilization Review on Hospital Use and Expenditures: A Review of the Literature and an Update on Recent Findings," *Medical Care Review*, 47(3):327–363, Fall 1990.

Williams, R. B., J. C. Barefoot, R. M. Califf, et al., "Prognostic Importance of Social and Economic Resources Among Medically Treated Patients with Angiographically Documented Coronary Artery Disease," *JAMA*, 267(4):520–524, 1992.

Yin, R. K., *Case Study Research: Design and Methods* (2nd ed.), Thousand Oaks, CA: Sage Publications, 1994.

Yusuf, S., et al., "Beta Blockage During and After Myocardial Infarction: An Overview of the Randomized Trials," *Progress in Cardiovascular Diseases*, 27:335–371, 1985.

Yusuf, S., J. Wittes, and L. Friedman, "Overview of Results of Randomized Clinical Trials in Heart Disease: I. Treatments Following Myocardial Infarction," *JAMA*, 260:2088–2093, 1988.

Zwanziger, J., G. A. Melnick, and A. Bamezai, "Costs and Price Competition in California Hospitals, 1980–1990," *Health Affairs*, 13(4):118–126, Fall 1994.

Accreditation | Formal process by which an authorized body assesses and recognizes an organization, a program, a group, or an individual as complying with established standards or criteria.

Acute disease | A disease having a rapid onset and lasting for a short time, such as fewer than 30 days (e.g., cold or flu). Compare: chronic disease.

Administrative data | Information on the utilization of and charges for services maintained by insurance companies and other payors. See: claims data.

Alternative hypothesis | The alternative to the null hypothesis. Usually corresponds to the presence of the effect being investigated. Often is denoted as H_A or H_1. Compare: null hypothesis.

Ambulatory care | Medical care provided to a patient without hospitalization, generally in an office or clinic.

Analysis of covariance (ANOCOVA) | A statistical model used to examine the variation in a continuous dependent variable that is explained by a group of independent variables that are qualitative and continuous. This method combines standard linear regression and ANOVA.

Analysis of variance (ANOVA) | A statistical model used to examine how much of the variation in a continuous dependent variable is explained by qualitative (categorical) independent variable(s). See: F-statistic.

Appropriateness of care	A performance dimension evaluating whether the health benefits expected from a medical intervention exceed the expected health risks by a sufficient margin that the intervention is worth doing.
Baseline data	An observation or measurement that represents the starting level, generally used for comparison purposes after some intervention has been given or time has elapsed.
Beneficiary	A person eligible to receive benefits from an insurance policy, a health care financing program (e.g., Medicare or Medicaid), or a prepaid health plan (e.g., HMO).
Bias	A systematic error in data resulting from the methods, tools, or environment of data collection and processing (i.e., nonrandom error).
Capitation	A system of payment for health services where the health plan or provider is paid a fixed fee for each enrollee and is responsible for providing services for that fee.
Case mix	Refers to the distribution of patients by categories such as age, gender, disease, severity of illness, etc.; case mix factors are often cited as reasons for differences in health care spending
Causal inference	Judgments about cause and effect relationships, as between poisoning and sickness.
Chronic disease	A disease or illness that lasts a long time, such as months or years (e.g., asthma or high blood pressure). Compare: acute disease.
Claims data	Data collected by insurance companies to determine eligibility and level of payment for services rendered.
COBRA '85	Consolidated Omnibus Budget Reconciliation Act of 1985. Federal legislation that instituted a number of consumer protections. One widely known provision relates to allowing continued access to employer-sponsored group health coverage for 18 months after employment has ended.

Coding conventions System for assigning a number or other symbol as a substitute for a more extensive item of information (e.g., diagnosis codes or procedure codes).

Coefficient of variation (COV) A statistical measure of the relative variability around a mean; it is calculated by dividing the standard deviation by the mean.

Commercial insurer Generally used to refer to employer-based insurance coverage.

Comorbid condition A disease or condition present at the same time as the principal disease or condition of a patient.

Conceptual framework Provides structure to the study of a problem by organizing the factors that may contribute to the problem.

Confidence interval A range of possible parameter values constructed from the observed data using statistical theory. A confidence interval takes into account the uncertainty of the estimate that is due to sampling. A confidence interval always has an associated confidence level (e.g., 95 percent). See: parameter, confidence level.

Confidence level A statistical quantity representing the degree to which the researcher believes that the confidence interval contains the population parameter of interest. A common confidence interval is 95 percent. If repeated samples were taken from the population that percentage (e.g., 95 percent) of confidence intervals would contain the true population parameter on average. See: confidence interval, parameter, sample.

Consistency A statistical concept describing a large-sample property. As the sample size increases, the estimator gets closer to the true value of the parameter.

Contingency table A two-dimensional table whose rows are defined by the categories of one variable, and whose columns are defined by the categories of another variable. A cell in the table contains the number (frequency) of observations that are found jointly in the row variable and associated column variable. Usually analyzed using a chi-square statistic. See: cross-tabulation.

Continuous variable	A quantitative variable with no gaps between possible values (e.g., blood pressure values). Compare: discrete variable.
Continuously enrolled	Enrolled in a health plan for a specified period without any breaks in coverage.
Convenience sample	Individuals or groups selected for study because of convenience factors (e.g., time, location, or access). Not randomly selected and therefore not representative of the general population.
Copayment	A form of patient cost-sharing in which a fixed sum or percentage of the bill is paid by the insured person for each health service. Compare: deductible.
Cost-benefit ratio	A mathematical quantity that represents the net benefit per unit of cost for a specific activity. Used to compare different activities/projects (benefits ÷ costs).
Cost-effective	An analysis used to determine which intervention achieves the greatest benefit for a fixed level of total expenditures.
Covariate	Independent variable in a regression model.
Coverage exclusions	Types of medical care and procedures specifically excluded from insurance coverage, such as for experimental treatments.
CPT code	A code from the Physician's Current Procedural Terminology (CPT) (published by the American Medical Association). A systematic listing and coding of procedures and services.
Cross-sectional data	Information on an item of interest (e.g., patient) collected or measured at *a given point in time.*
Cross-tabulation	A statistical table that illustrates the relationship between two variables by showing the frequency with which combinations of values occur. See: contingency table.
Data repository	A place where data from many different sources are collected and stored.

Data base	An organized collection of information, data, and text stored in a standardized and accessible format.
Deductible	A form of cost-sharing where a set amount must be paid by the patient before any payments are made by the insurer. Compare: copayment.
Demographic characteristics	Characteristics that describe a person or population, such as age, gender, race, income, and education.
Dependent variable	The outcome of interest or response that you want to understand. Often denoted as the "y" variable.
Diagnosis code	A numerical system for classifying diseases, conditions, and injuries (e.g., International Classification of Diseases, Ninth Revision [ICD-9-CM] codes).
Diagnosis related groups (DRGs)	A method for classifying Medicare patients by the expected resources to be utilized in treating them. Used to formulate the reimbursement rate made to hospitals under the Prospective Payment System.
Discrete variable	A quantitative variable where gaps exist between the possible values. It can assume only a finite or countable number of distinct values (e.g., the number of medical visits). Compare: continuous variable.
Disease severity	The degree or state of seriousness of a patient's disease.
Effectiveness	Degree to which a health care intervention achieves desired outcomes under usual care conditions. Consideration of cost is not required.
Efficacy	The degree to which the intervention has been shown to achieve the desired effect, result, or objective under ideal circumstances (e.g., application of treatment in an experimental study).
Efficiency	Relationship between the outcomes and the resources used to deliver care to achieve the outcome.
Eligibility data	Data used to determine whether a person can be reinbursed under a health insurance plan. See: enrollment data.

Encounter data	Information about or resulting from a contact between a patient and a health care provider. Contains information on costs and services used. See: administrative data.
Enhanced enrollment data	In addition to basic enrollment data, enrollment files ideally should also contain unique patient and dependent identifiers, demographic and employment information, plan information, health status information, and at least quarterly updating. See: enrollment data.
Enrollment data	Data on enrolled subscribers of a health insurance plan; the data contain information such as the name of the policyholder, type of coverage, and enrollment date.
Episode of care	A sequence of care by a hospital or physician for a specific medical problem or condition, from onset to resolution of the problem.
F-statistic	A statistical hypothesis test that utilizes a probability distribution called an F-distribution, which is calculated using the ratio of two independent random variables with chi-squared distributions. F-tests are important in performing an analysis of variance (ANOVA). See: analysis of variance
Fee-for-service (FFS) plan	A method of paying physicians and other health care providers for each service or encounter (for example, a doctor's office visit or an operation).
Financial incentive	A monetary reward to motivate behavior.
Focus group	A method for generating information or testing how people will respond to a message/product. A small number of individuals are brought together in a group and, under the leadership of a facilitator, asked to express their opinions on some topic.
Frequency	The count of the number of observations that have a particular value for the variable of interest.
Functional status	A measure of an individual's ability to perform various physical, mental, and social activities (e.g., Activities of Daily Living).

Health care delivery system	A term that refers to all the facilities and services, along with methods for financing them, through which health care is provided.
Health maintenance organization (HMO)	A health care organization that acts as both the insurer and provider of medical services. Services are provided on a capitated basis (fixed amount per person or per service).
Health plan	An organization that provides a specific set of medical, hospital, and related services to individuals or contracts with other organizations to provide these services to a group of subscribers.
Health status	A measure of an individual's state of health (e.g., poor, fair, good, or excellent).
Healthy People 2000	A U.S. Department of Health and Human Services document that outlines a set of national health objectives to be accomplished by the year 2000. The objectives focus on the prevention of disease and promotion of health at a community level.
Histogram	A graphical representation of a frequency table.
Hospice program	A program that assists with the physical, emotional, spiritual, psychological, social, financial, and legal needs of the dying patient and his or her family.
Iatrogenic injury	Illness or injury resulting from health care delivery (i.e., nosocomial infections). Example: infections acquired from the hospital stay.
ICD-9-CM code	International Classification of Diseases, Ninth Revision. The codes are used to classify diagnoses and procedures, primarily for reimbursement purposes.
Impute missing data	An analytic technique that involves assigning values to missing data.
Incidence rate	The fraction of a population that is newly diagnosed with a condition within a specified time frame.

Independent practice association (IPA)	A name for a health maintenance organization that contracts with physicians usualy in solo or small group practices. The physicians maintain their own practices but agree to furnish services to patients who are enrolled in a prepaid plan in which the physician services are supplied at a fixed cost to the enrollee. See: capitation.
Independent variable	The factor that influences or is related to the dependent variable or outcome. Independent variables are sometimes called covariates or predictor variables, and are often denoted as "x" variables.
Indication	A guideline or rule that specifies when certain medical interventions are necessary or appropriate.
Indicator	A quantitative measure used to improve the performance of functions, processes, and outcomes.
Inference	Judgments or deductions about a set of facts, based on observation or experimentation.
Internal consistency checks	Checks to monitor whether all of the data for an individual are in agreement.
Interquartile range	The difference between the 75th and 25th percentiles.
Intervention	An action taken with the intent to change the present condition or interrupt the flow of events.
Longitudinal data	Data that record the behavior of interest on the same individuals or facilities *over time*. Repeated measures of a single sample in different periods of time.
Managed care	A term used to refer more generally to systems in which services are provided for a fixed fee. Often used as a synonym for health maintenance organization.
Market area	The geographical region in which a health care provider or organization sells its services.
Mean	The arithmetic average, or the sum of all values divided by the number of observations with values.
Median	The midpoint of the data; 50 percent of the values are higher than the median and 50 percent are lower than the median.

Medicaid	The federal program established in 1965 that provides health care to poor women and children, the disabled, and the poor elderly. The program is jointly funded with the states.
Medical record	An account of a patient's medical history, including illness, treatments, examination results, test results, notes, and conclusions.
Medicare	A federal program established in 1965 that provides health care to persons age 65 and older and to others entitled to Social Security benefits (i.e., disabled).
Mode	The most frequently observed value.
Morbidity	The presence of a disease or illness that affects the individual's ability to function.
Mortality	Death.
Multiple linear regression	A statistical model with more than one independent variable that is linear in the coefficients. This model may be appropriate when several independent variables are likely to simultaneously affect the dependent variable, and when the dependent variable is continuous.
Multiple logistic regression	A statistical model that is conceptually similar to multiple linear regression and is used when the dependent variable is binary (i.e., can take on only two values, such as yes/no) rather than continuous. The independent variables may be qualitative or continuous.
Nominal variable	Qualitative variable where no natural ordering to the values or categories exists.
Nonresponse	Used in survey research to refer to the situation of persons who do not answer surveys or who do not answer particular questions on surveys.
Nonresponse weights	Quantities used in analysis to re-weight survey results to take into account the fact that some individuals sampled did not respond.

Null hypothesis	The statistical hypothesis, or mathematical statement about the population parameter, that is being tested for possible rejection. Usually corresponds to an absence of the effect being investigated. Often is denoted as H_0. See: Type I and Type II errors. Compare: alternative hypothesis.
Odds ratio	A frequently used means to express the relative effect of the independent variable on the dependent variable in a logistic regression model. If the odds ratio for a particular independent variable is less than one, this indicates that the odds that the dependent variable occurs decrease with higher values of the independent variable. If the odds ratio is greater than one, this indicates that the odds of the independent variable occurring increase with higher values of the independent variable. See: multiple logistic regression.
Open enrollment	A limited time period, usually occurring annually, during which individuals are given the opportunity to change health care plans.
Ordinal variable	Qualitative variable where a natural ordering to the values or categories exists. The intervals between values are not meaningful for ordinal variables.
Out-of-range values	Numbers that are not reasonable values for the variable in question.
Parameter	A statistical quantity representing the actual, or "true," summary measure for the entire population of interest.
P-value	The probability (p) value measures of a hypothesis test. A statistical quantity for the probability of getting a result as extreme or more extreme than that actually observed, given that the null hypothesis is true.
Population	The entire group of people, facilities, or items that meet a condition; for example, all people who reside in a defined geographic area (e.g., residents of Dallas) or individuals who meet a certain description (e.g., the uninsured).
Population subgroup	A subset of a larger population group. Example: Population is all citizens of the United States; subgroup is all women in the United States.

Power analysis	Used to estimate the sample size required to detect a difference or change of interest using a statistical hypothesis test.
Power of a test	Equal to the probability of rejecting the null hypothesis when it is false, or one minus the probability of a Type II error. See: null hypothesis, Type II error.
Practical difference	A difference large enough to have clinical or policy relevance.
Practice guidelines	Standards for clinical approaches to medical conditions or diseases that specify care for the typical patient in a typical situation.
Pre-existing health condition	A physical or mental condition that has been discovered before an individual applies for health insurance.
Precision analysis	A statistical technique to determine the sample size required to construct a confidence interval of certain length. See: confidence interval, confidence level, standard deviation.
Predictors	Factors that are used in models to explain variation in an important outcome. See: covariate, independent variable.
Preferred provider organization (PPO)	A pre-negotiated arrangement between providers (hospitals and doctors) and purchasers (insurers) to furnish health services to a group of patients. Fee discounts are negotiated in return for guaranteed patient volume. Patients may obtain services outside the PPO network of providers but typically pay more to use out-of-network providers.
Premium	A payment required for an insurance policy for a given period of time.
Prevalence rate	The fraction of a population having a disease, condition, or attribute of interest at a particular point in time. Compare: incidence rate.
Preventive care	Care designed to prevent disease or injury from occurring.
Primary care	Basic health care that emphasizes treatment for common illnesses and injuries.

Primary diagnosis	A judgment about the most likely disease or condition affecting a patient's health.
Private purchaser	A nongovernment entity that purchases insurance or health services (e.g., employers or consumers).
Probability sample	A randomly drawn subset of individuals from a population in which each individual has a known probability of being sampled.
Procedure code	A system for classifying medical services and procedures (e.g., CPT-4 codes).
Process of care	The interaction between individuals and health care providers that results in the utilization of services.
Prospective data collection	Data collection planned in anticipation of an event or occurrence.
Prospective payment system (PPS)	The pricing system currently used to pay for hospital services provided to Medicare patients. Payments are based on classifying patients by DRGs.
Provider	A hospital, health care institution, or health care professional that provides health care services to patients.
Proxy measure	A substitute measure.
Public domain	Freely available to the public; not privately held or owned; nonproprietary.
Public health program	A program created to improve the health of the community.
Qualitative variable	Variable with values that do not lie on a numeric scale. Qualitative variables also may be referred to as categorical variables. See: ordinal variable and nominal variable.
Quality assessment	Measurement and analysis of the quality of care provided to groups or individuals.
Quantitative variable	Variable with values that lie on a numeric scale. See: discrete variable and continuous variable.
Quota sample	A sample resulting from a method that selects individuals/hospitals based on achieving a target number or proportion of persons with certain characteristics.

Example: If half of the population is to be composed of persons over age 50, then people will be enrolled in the study until the target proportion has been achieved (nonrandom; nonprobability-based sampling approach).

Random sample	A sample resulting from a method that allows each person/facility an equal chance of being selected. Probability-based sampling approach.
Range	The difference between the maximum and minimum values. Compare: interquartile range.
Rate	The frequency with which an event occurs in a defined population per unit of time or per number of possible occurrences. Example: If 100 children receive DPT immunizations out of 1,000 eligible children, then the rate is 100/1,000 = 0.10 (10 percent).
Registry	A data base containing information on a particular topic, such as birth defects or tumors.
Regression coefficients	Statistical estimates in a regression model of the direction and magnitude of the association between each independent variable, or covariate, and the outcome when all other factors are held constant.
Reliability	Consistency in the results of a measure. Tendency of the measure to produce the same result twice.
Report card	A periodic report on the quality or cost of services. Used to share information with providers or consumers.
Response rate	In surveys, the percentage of persons/facilities given questionnaires who complete and return them.
Retrospective data collection	Data collection for events that have already occurred; going back in time.
Risk factor	A factor that increases one's chances of contracting a disease or dying. Examples: Smoking is a risk factor for lung cancer; high blood pressure is a risk factor for coronary heart disease.

Risk adjustment | A way to "correct" for differences in patient characteristics that may influence the outcome of care, independent from medical treatment. The process uses severity-of-illness measures such as age, gender, and presence of comorbid conditions to adjust a patient's risk of mortality or morbidity.

Sample | A subgroup drawn from a larger population that can be used to construct estimates of events in the whole population. The size of the sample is usually denoted as "n." See also: random sample.

Sampling weight | A statistical quantity usually equal to the inverse of the probability of being sampled and used in analysis to infer from the sample to the population.

Secondary data analysis | Use of already collected data to study a problem.

Secondary diagnosis | Any medical condition other than the primary diagnosis that exists at the time of hospital admission or that develops subsequently and affects the treatment the patient receives.

Sequelae | The after-effect of disease or injury; a secondary result.

Severity adjustment | A way to "correct" for differences in the seriousness of a particular illness that may affect comparisons of health outcomes. For example, the severity of angina and hypertension have been defined and standardized.

Severity of illness | The level or extent of disease in a patient.

Simple random sample | Sample in which every member of the population has an equal probability of being selected.

Standard error | A statistical quantity equal to the standard deviation divided by the square root of the sample size; measures the error in a mean (average).

Standard deviation | A statistical quantity equal to the square root of the average squared distance between each value and the mean.

Standardization | To conform to a standard (e.g., convert everything to the same units for comparison purposes).

Statistically significant	A test statistic that is as large or larger than a predetermined requirement. Results in the rejection of the null hypothesis. A statistically significant observed difference is determined to be unlikely to occur by chance with a predetermined significance level (e.g., 5 percent).
Surveillance	Ongoing monitoring to detect changes in trend or distribution (e.g., AIDS surveillance).
Survey data	Data collected from individuals (e.g., patients) or organizations (e.g., hospitals or insurers) that often are used to study special issues not captured in routine data collection such as encounter data.
T-test	A statistic computed from the sample and used to evaluate whether differences between means (averages) are likely to have occured by chance.
Type I error	A type of statistical error that arises if the null hypothesis is rejected when it is true. The probability of Type I error is usually denoted as α. See: null hypothesis.
Type II error	A type of statistical error that arises if the null hypothesis is not rejected when it is false. The probability of Type II error is usually denoted as β. See: null hypothesis.
Universal coverage	The provision of health insurance coverage to all citizens.
Upcoding	Coding a medical service, procedure, or diagnosis to obtain a higher payment for services rendered. When payment is based on the patient diagnosis code (e.g., ICD-9-CM), as is the case for hospital payment under the PPS, then "upcoding" refers to a diagnosis code selection that may not reflect the actual clinical scenario. When payment is based on the medical service or procedure code (e.g., CPT-4), then "upcoding" typically refers to a service or procedure code.

| Utilization review | The examination and evaluation of the necessity, appropriateness, and efficacy of the use of health services (e.g., review of appropriateness of admissions and length of stay). |
| Validity | Degree to which an item accurately measures what it intends to measure. |

SOURCES USED TO COMPLETE GLOSSARY:

Aday, Lu Ann, Charles E. Begley, David R. Lairson, and Carl H. Slater, *Evaluating the Medical Care System: Effectiveness, Efficiency, Equity*, Ann Arbor, MI: Health Administration Press, 1993.

American Hospital Association booklet, "Transforming Health Care Delivery," 1994.

Banus, D., K. Kunz, and T. Macdonald, *Health Care Reform*, Berkeley, CA: Institute of Governmental Studies Press, U.C. Berkeley, 1994.

Cochran, W. G., *Sampling Techniques* (3rd ed.), New York: John Wiley & Sons, 1977.

Health Insurance Association of America, *Source Book of Health Insurance Data*, Washington, DC, 1994.

Koutsoyiannis, A., *Theory of Econometrics: An Introductory Exposition of Econometric Methods* (2nd ed.), London: The MacMillan Press Ltd., 1985.

Last, J. M., *A Dictionary of Epidemiology* (2nd ed.), New York: Oxford University Press, Inc., 1988.

Mansfield, E., *Statistics for Business and Economics: Methods and Applications*, Fourth Edition, New York: W. W. Norton and Company, 1991.

O'Leary, M. R., et al., *Lexikon: Dictionary of Health Care Terms, Organizations, and Acronyms for the Era of Reform*, Oakbrook Terrace, IL: Joint Commission on Accreditation of Healthcare Organizations, 1994.

Slee, V., and D. Slee, *Health Care Reform Terms* (2nd ed.), St. Paul, MN: Tringa Press, 1994.

Stokey, E., and R. Zeckhauser, *A Primer for Policy Analysis*, New York: W. W. Norton and Company, 1978.

Thomas, C. L., *Taber's Cyclopedic Medical Dictionary*, Edition 15, Philadelphia, PA: F. A. Davis Company, 1981.

Weisberg, H. F., and B. D. Bowen, *An Introduction to Survey Research and Data Analysis*, San Francisco, CA: W. H. Freeman and Co., 1977.

INDEX

Elizabeth A. McGlynn, Ph.D., Director, RAND Health Center for Research on Quality in Health Care, is a nationally known expert in measurement of quality of care.

Cheryl L. Damberg, Ph.D., is Director of Research and Quality at the Pacific Business Group on Health.

Eve A. Kerr, M.D., M.P.H., is a Research Investigator at the Ann Arbor Veterans Affairs Center for Practice Management and Outcomes Research, and Assistant Professor of Medicine, University of Michigan School of Medicine.

Robert H. Brook, M.D., Sc.D., F.A.C.P., is Vice President and Director of RAND Health and Professor of Medicine and Health Services at the UCLA Center for Health Sciences. Dr. Brook has an international reputation for his work on appropriateness and quality of care.